MW01614037

D

and
BARBED WIRE:
A CANCER CRUSADE

© ASHCO PUBLICATIONS, INC.

ISBN: 0-9661937-4-1

Printed in the United States of America

FIRST EDITION

ASHCO PUBLICATIONS, INC.
P.O. Box 3066
Ashtabula, OH 44005-3066
(E-mail to: ashco@apk.net)
Fax: 440-964-5967

i

A PERCENTAGE OF PROFITS WILL BE DONATED TO THE FOLLOWING CHARITABLE ORGANIZATIONS

Regional Cancer Center, Erie, PA
(In memory of author's cousin, Jane Grady,
whose crusade ended in January, 2001)

St. Brigid's Church, Meadville, PA
(Building and Maintenance Fund)

Mind and Body Wellness Center
Meadville, PA

Family House, Pittsburgh, PA 15213
(Cindi Roth, Executive Director)
(In memory of a dear friend, Betty Dunbar,
whose crusade ended in February, 2001)

Visiting Nurse Association of Crawford
County, Meadville, PA

ABOUT THE TITLE

As the reader will come to learn, I have become quite involved in gardening in the past 18 months. Both my wife and I reside in a rural setting on an acre of land, which still has evidence of old fencing with barbed wire. One particular day, I was attempting to transplant some wild daisies when I came upon a "clump" that had grown through some rusty and corroded pieces of barbed wire, which were previously part of a fence. As I studied this mixture, I came to a conclusion that many of our days over the past 18 months were very much like daisies and barbed wire. In addition, some days were a mixture of both. More importantly, however, both continued to survive and so did we.

SPECIAL THANKS TO:

Mary Z. Burchard—Designer of Cover

Joy "J.D." Dunbar—Photograph
CEO, R.U.L.E.
Rural Leadership Program
Penn State University

iii

CONTENTS

CONTENTS

Page

DEDICATIONS

- To Eleanore Kudlawiec, my mother, who has lived a life with grace, a special touch of class and an undaunting courage through a lifetime of adversity.

- To Jane Grady, my cousin, whose courage in her 5 year battle against cancer has been nothing short of an inspiration.

- To Joy "J.D." Dunbar, a dear friend, who has always been there for both my wife and me. She may not be able to "sing," but she knows how to "soothe."

- To Dr. LeAnn Chrisman, Primary Care Physician for both my wife and me. Her ability and quickness to diagnose our medical conditions has extended both of our lives (if she hasn't saved them).

- To Chris Palotas, my loving wife, whose tenacity, advocacy, hope, faith and love brought me from the edge of death and despair to the threshold of a special freedom of spirit and the true knowledge of what love is "both in sickness and in health."

vi

SPECIAL RECOGNITION

I give a special salute to all my fellow cancer patients, who fight the battle on a daily basis.

My concern in this area is that after a number of years when the patient is "cancer-free," he/she is referred to as a "cancer survivor." I, personally, abhor that description because it implies that the patient has played a passive, re-active role in their treatment.

As a patient, I believe we should be referred to as "cancer crusaders" for several reasons. Namely, crusader implies the following characteristics: pro-active, aggressive, positive, willing to take chances, willing to fight for a "heavenly cause," ongoing willingness to continue the fight—because whether it's 1 year, 5 years or whatever—the crusade goes on!!

CHAPTER 1

Prologue To Pandemonium

October, 1996 to July, 1998

LIFE WAS GOOD... In October, 1996, my wife, Chris, and I celebrated our 25th anniversary. Earlier that year, I had encountered two incidents of rectal bleeding. However, after several tests, it was determined that I was suffering from ulcerative colitis. A regimen of diet and medication would control this situation.

LIFE WAS GOOD.... Both my wife and I were happy and content in our own professions—she as a social worker and I as an assistant district manager for a rehabilitation and social service agency for the blind and visually impaired.

LIFE WAS GOOD... In March of 1998, I began to display some signs of weight loss, appetite changes, thirst, sweating and so on. It would be determined that I had type II diabetes. Luckily, for me, this would and could be controlled by diet and exercise.

LIFE WAS GOOD.... During this same period, my wife began to display a number of symptoms. Basically, she had uncontrolled high blood pressure, as well as, type II diabetes. It appeared that any numerous combination of medications was not working. Additionally, over time, her physician determined other symptoms that were not as evident. She displayed what would be called a "Buffalo Hump" on the back of her neck, truncular obesity, irregular menstrual cycles, a sluggishness, some shortness of breath while walking stairs, and a history of difficulty getting pregnant.

Her physician, Dr. LeAnn Chrisman, (and mine as well) began to put all these things together. She ordered some tests and it would be confirmed that Chris had a "pituitary adenoma." In the simplest of terms, a tumor on the pituitary gland, which is located at the base of the brain.

Both she and I went to Pittsburgh Allegheny General Hospital, where we met with a number of specialists to confirm the diagnosis and review options. The bottom line was that it was a "pituitary adenoma" and had to come out.

After reviewing several options and speaking with other patients, a decision was made in June that Chris would have surgery on July 22, 1998.

LIFE WAS GOOD... History showed that 95% of these tumors were benign. The official term for this is "Cushing's Disease."

LIFE WAS GOOD... Between May and July, 1998, I had undergone two vigorous interviews for the position of Director of Field Operations for the Bureau of Blindness and Visual Services. In fact, I was the successful candidate, had been appointed to the position and would begin after Chris's surgery. I would take up residency part of the time in Harrisburg. PA—the state capitol—and spend weekends at home. *LIFE WAS still GOOD...*

During this same period, I continued to display a weight loss and lack of appetite. In addition, my urine became dark. I placed these symptoms in the arena of diabetes. Unfortunately, I also began to display a yellowish tinting of my skin. In fact, the whites of my eyes seemed somewhat yellow.

When I returned from Harrisburg, my wife convinced me that I needed to see my physician; especially, if I was going to take up residency in Harrisburg. *LIFE WAS still GOOD...*

Chris was able to get me an appointment for Friday, July 17, 1998, at 10:00 a.m. *LIFE WAS GOOD!!!*

CHAPTER 2

The Big Exam

10:00 a.m. Friday, July 17, 1998...

Not much time was spent in the waiting room. Chris accompanied me as she wasn't sure I'd share all information I might have gathered. My doctor was on time and not running late that day — maybe because it was Friday. As I sat on the examining table, both my wife and I explained my ongoing symptoms. My eyes and skin were studied for some time.

Next, I was asked to lie down so that an exam could be done to check my organs—basically, kidneys, stomach, liver, and those adjacent areas. The exam was done. *LIFE WAS GOOD....*

10:45 a.m.

As we stepped out of the exam room, one physician explained she wanted some additional tests done. It would require me to drink one jug of a wonderful white "chalky" substance before I left the office. I could take the second jug home, consume three-fourths of it, return to the hospital for a CAT scan test and consume the remainder of the "afternoon cocktail." The test was scheduled for 1:00 p.m.

1:15 p.m.

I waited outside the testing area and in fact, tried to give up my jug to another patient—unfortunately, no luck! The test itself took less than a half an hour and was uneventful. I returned home to get some rest. *LIFE WAS GOOD....*

*LIFE WAS GOOD...*My wife and I were scheduled to attend a wedding that evening some 45 miles north of our home. It was a beautiful evening ceremony and reception. It was a busy weekend, we were scheduled to attend another family wedding reception Saturday afternoon.

Another beautiful day—another beautiful event. It was great to see so many family members and friends in such a short time span—*LIFE WAS INDEED GOOD!!!*

Sunday, July 19, 1998—A day of rest.

CHAPTER 3

Diagnosis, Prognosis, Treatment

9:00 a.m. Monday, July 20, 1998

As planned, I was to return to my physician's office in the hope that test results would be completed and we could determine what needed to be done. My wife and I were escorted to an examining room. As before, my weight, blood pressure, and temperature were taken. We waited patiently (no pun intended) for my physician to appear.

A knock came at the door and Dr. Chrisman appeared. She stated that we needed to come with her to her office. My heart began to race. As I walked through the hall to her office, I noticed that other staff people were not looking at us. It was as if we didn't exist. My stomach began to sink and rumble. Something in my gut began to tell me, maybe life isn't so good after all!!

My physician began to go over test results—everything showed up during the scan as normal, except there appeared to be a growth on my pancreas. In the simplest of terms, the reading and interpretation of the test revealed that I had pancreatic cancer.

My wife began to weep. My physician cradled her in her arms, as tears began to well up in her eyes as well.

I stood in position, not moving, maybe not even breathing. I was stunned! I was mesmerized! I felt mummified! A huge warmth took over the interior of my body as if I was on fire. I was horrified! I was in a catatonic state! I couldn't speak! What the X!?#X! is happening to me? I was scared to death—the one thing I had always told my wife about death was that I could deal with anything, but I didn't want to die because of cancer. My wife hugged me. My doctor hugged me. They both shed tears while I stood there in a stupefied trance. *LIFE WAS GOOD*....my ass!!

I quickly learned more about medicine, more about cancer, more about the pancreas, more about pancreatic cancer than I ever wanted to know. This is not a good cancer to have. If you have a chance to choose a cancer—leave this one out of the selection pool.

My physician began to explain options. She advised me that she had made an appointment for me to see a surgeon and specialist in gastro-enterology. His office was located at Presbyterian Hospital in Pittsburgh, PA. My appointment was for 3:00 p.m. today. She insisted I had to have someone other than my wife or me drive to this appointment. I would need to take all my test results and medical records with me.

While in the doctor's office, my wife called a friend, Judy Kirberger, who worked in the same building. She later joined us in the doctor's office for support. The doctor insisted there was no way we were to drive to Pittsburgh by ourselves. My wife then called another couple, Mark and Renate Stellato, who were our friends. She explained the situation and a plan was developed that we would ride in our friend's van and leave by 12:30 p.m.

8

We still had to get home, contact our son, explain the situation as best we could, determine if he could/would come with us and so on.

11:00 a.m.

We left the doctor's office with pamphlets explaining services at Presbyterian Hospital, the University of Pittsburgh School of Medicine, the Cancer Institute at Montefiore Hospital, directions on how to get where and so on. We had something to eat (I think), and my wife contacted our son, who was able to get out of work to join us.

12:30 p.m.

We had about enough time to catch our breath, when our son and friends arrived and we were on our way. I would serve as navigator. Bad Mistake! As it turned out, I got us lost—who knows, maybe it was on purpose. Anyway, we arrived. *LIFE WAS GOOD?*

2:30 p.m.

Having arrived at the correct office, much time was spent gathering personal and insurance data. Next, I was weighed, and blood pressure and temperature were taken.

My wife, son and I were escorted to an examination room, where we were met by a medical student, who was specifically assigned to this physician. He would spend some time gathering information as to how and what caused us to get to this point. We were advised that we

9

would next be seen by the surgeon, DR. WOLFGANG SCHROAT!!! "Oh, my God!" I thought. "I hope he didn't attend Heinrich Hemler's School of Surgery."

Dr. Schroat was not a large man, had a slight build, somewhat bald with graying hair. He definitely had a German accent. He performed an exam by feeling my organs and reviewing the scans. He confirmed that this definitely appeared to be pancreatic cancer. He explained what they could do.

They would take me into surgery and go through my navel and determine (by camera) if anything could be done. If something could be done, they would perform what is known as the "Whipple Procedure." In the simplest of terms, they would remove whatever portion of the pancreas was affected by the growth. They would remove parts of any organs directly in contact with the pancreatic tumor.

This could have an impact on numerous organs and could take some time. Another thing, I needed to make a decision today as to what and when I want to do this, as Dr. Schroat would be going to Europe in the next two weeks. He did not want to leave in the middle of my treatment. The bottom line was simply this—you need this procedure done and you need it done now—sooner not later.

I made the decision on the spot. The surgery would occur on Friday, July 24, 1998. I would be in Pittsburgh on most of Thursday for pre-operation work-ups and tests. I had just decided to allow someone I spoke with for twenty minutes to perhaps spend hours inside my body—trying to save my life.

10

4:15 p.m.

We left Pittsburgh on a somewhat uneventful trip back home. We stopped for dinner at a Bob Evans Restaurant. The least I could do is pay for gas and dinner. My only question is which came first. The trip home was quiet and somber.

Tuesday, July 21, 1998

The day was spent making phone calls--my wife to her mother, me to my parents. My wife called her surgeon in Pittsburgh to advise that she had to postpone her surgery until sometime after mine. I had to call my current boss and my secretary to explain the situation, the planned surgery and so on.

It was also necessary to be "patched through" to Harrisburg so I could speak to the agency director. I had to advise him that I must withdraw my name from my recent appointment as field operations director. I had some other pressing assignment that was going to take up a great deal of my time.

Wednesday, July 22, 1998

Most of the day was spent talking with friends and relatives, who had already gotten the word by the grapevine. It was somewhat of an introspective day for both my wife and myself. It was a day filled with tears.

LIFE WAS GOOD... Well, yes, it had been.

7:00 a.m.
Thursday, July 23, 1998

This was the day scheduled to return to Pittsburgh for pre-operation work ups. I spent most of the morning walking in a daze, into the walls or into my wife. The plan was that we would leave for Pittsburgh by 8:30 a.m. so that I could get to the hospital for tests. We would be spending the evening at a "Family House" supported by the hospital system. It also would provide bus shuttle service to and from the hospital.

Early that morning I would write a letter to my wife with an additional enclosure written on November 4. 1997. That date was around the time we completed our wills, living wills, and power of attorneys. As I write this, I have just opened that envelope and have seen it for the first time.

July 23, 1998

My Dear Wife,

If you are at the point of reading this, I don't have to explain where I am—you get the picture.

It indeed has been a "fun run" and being with you has made it so. We "complete" each other and in all of this, you have played a large role in any successes I may have achieved. I want to share some last thoughts and wishes with you.

12

What to do:

I'd like to be buried out of Mizner's place with a wood casket. Pall Bearers: Butch & Bud, Bob Pears, Mike Koncewicz, Clark Bryant and Andy Stofan.

Let Butryn do the mass with burial at either St. Hippolyte's or St. Brigid's cemetery.

Ask the following to do eulogies after the mass: Msgr. "Max" Karg to discuss my faith in God, and in self, others, church. Bob Lamb to discuss my hope for everyone and BVS. J.D. to discuss my love for all. (I have enclosed other funeral instructions.)

Life Insurance:

Between IDS, State Farm and State Employee Life insurance, there is more than enough to cover this house, the car and credit card loan. There should be about $30,000.00 from vacation and sick leave to cover other funeral expenses. Getting my lump sum retirement and investing it should put you in good shape.

The Apartment House:

Please consider "deeding" it to Scott and Sharon. You need to rid yourself of this responsibility and maybe this will teach him some. You may need to give him some money for roof repairs. Ultimately, this will be your decision.

I think that essentially deals with financial issues.

Back to pallbearers, others can be named as honorary ones. I just tried to avoid slighting any of our friends, but , again the final call will be yours.

13

My parents:
Tell my mother I love her dearly and that she has always been an inspiration to me. Tell my father that I have grown to love him as such and thank him for bringing love and happiness to my mother's life. Watch out for them.
Your mom:
Tell her that while we never developed a warm relationship, I love her for producing you. Ask her to seize the moment, to renew, revitalize and rebuild her relationship with you as a daughter and with Scott as her only grandson.
Our families and friends:
I wanted to write to everyone, but time is of the essence. Extend my love and appreciation for them just being there throughout our lives.
In closing, be happy! Whatever you do, wherever you go—just be happy. Always remember me and the fun times. Forgive me for those times that weren't so good, but helped us through the learning process. (I forgot to tell you what I should be wearing—It's up to you—it's your last chance to do the "Ken Doll" thing.)
I love you! I truly love you all the days of my life and beyond!!! Finally, tell Scott and Sharon that I truly love them both and have only hopes for their best interests. Tell them to love one another and build on that love each day. He is truly a fine son and she will be a wonderful daughter. I remain his biggest fan!
Well, that's it. There probably could/should be more, but my head is spinning.

All my love,
George

14

November 4, 1997

To Whom It May Concern:

By the time you read this, I will be a part of history and in another place. With hope and prayer, one that is full of love, joy and laughter.

In any event, I want to leave instructions on how this celebration should occur—and I do mean <u>celebration</u>!! I want this to be a celebration of my life (marked by joy, hope and faith)—not a dirge of my death.

As a result, I want any church service to be uplifting and joyous. I have selected readings and music to be used during mass. They are as follows:

__Entrance Hymn__: "City of God"
(If the church permits the "Gloria" to be sung, let's do it!)

__First Reading__: First Letter of John 1 John 4:7-21 or Prophet Isaiah 6:1-8

__Responsorial Psalm__: Shepherd Me, O God! (sung, please!)

__Second Reading__: Paul's Second Letter to Timothy 2 Timothy 4: 6-8 or Romans 10:13-18

__Gospel__: John 14: 1-14 or 14: 23-29

__Offertory Songs__: "Be Not Afraid" <u>and</u> "On Eagle's Wings" (Two verses of each song)

__Communion__: "One Bread, One Body" <u>and</u> "Like a Shepherd" (Two verses of each song)

__Blessing at Casket__: Traditional "Farewell Song"

__Closing__: "We Remember" (All verses)

__Recessional from church__: Recording of "Amazing Grace," played on bagpipes. (This can be found at any local bagpipe store!)

15

In addition, before or after the blessing of the casket (whichever is more appropriate), anyone wishing to offer any remarks should be give that opportunity. Be nice!!

A last note—remember, this should be an uplifting and happy experience for all the participants. Don't let me down or I'll come back and cause havoc in your life.

Love you all,
George

P.S. Don't worry about the bagpipe music. My truly good friends (Hank and J.D) saw fit to meet my "bagpipe needs" before my time so that they could know that I would rest easy.

Love ya,
George

CHAPTER 4

Back In The Big City

8:30 a.m. Thursday, July 23, 1998

"It's off to see the Wizard—Because—Because—Because!"

The drive itself was uneventful. We arrived at the hospital and began the process.

First, we went for chest x-rays and found that everything was still in order and the surgery was still a "go."

Next, we went for blood work. Again, all systems appeared to be a "go."

Somehow, we squeezed lunch in, which would serve as my last food for the day.

We continued to move through the medical maze with the next stop being for the EKG. Apparently, I passed with flying colors. My last stop would be waiting to see the anesthesiologist.

This visit was somewhat unremarkable, as well. Measurements of my throat, neck and so on were taken. In addition, the attending physician felt my neck, throat and so on. He explained at great length what would transpire, how and when. He was unsure of the "who" except to say "…it won't be me, but it'll probably be a couple of people." In the last part of our conversation, he got a very serious look on his face. He said, "I must tell you some important information now. Before you sign any more papers; you need to know that you may not survive this surgery. I say that not to frighten you, but to make sure you understand the severity of this surgery and the ability of surviving."

"Thank you very much," I said. At least, I think that's what I said.

Next stop—pick up your liquid dinner for the rest of the evening. I swear whoever named these concoctions to clean out your colon are all out of work comedians. Imagine drinking something called "Bear Claw" or "Go Lightly."

Just my luck, I would get the latter. We then left the hospital and went to the "Family House." While there, I got to prepare the magic brew that would make me feel a special oneness with a white porcelain commode. The next twelve hours would, needless to say, be a moving experience.

In the room we shared, my son and his fiancé would sleep on air mattresses on the floor next to my wife, who slept in one of the twin beds. I would sleep (off and on) mostly off in the next twin bed. Interestingly enough, my bed would be the farthest from the bathroom. Whose bright idea was that?

4:00 a.m. Friday, July 24, 1998

I was up and completed my necessary tasks and woke up all the others. We needed to catch the shuttle bus at 4:45 a.m. as I had to be at the hospital at 5:00 a.m. Was this eternity or what?

5:00 a.m.

We arrived on time and I was escorted to a huge room. It was somewhat antiseptic in looks. It was surrounded by numerous curtains that were used to create cubicles and separate you from other patients. Of course, all my vitals were taken—still a "go!!"

I was instructed to take off all my clothing and put on this "half-assed gown." My clothes were taken to my family.

In the meantime, I was seen by three physicians, who would be monitoring the anesthesia. They checked my mouth and one remarked, that I needed some dental work. In response I stated I thought I had more important things to be concerned about besides my teeth. The three suggested that they place an epidural device that would subsequently be used to control pain. The suggestion was to do this while I was awake as it would be easier for everyone concerned. I consented to their request and all was still a "go!!"

It was approaching 6 to 6:30 a.m. and my family was escorted into my cubicle. This meeting (as I remember) lasted less than 5 minutes. My wife spoke to me and we kissed as I lay flat on a gurney. My son's fiancé (who is a nurse) wished me well and kissed me. Next my son, who was carrying my clothes and sneakers in a nylon sports bag bent over and kissed me for luck. Unfortunately, the nylon bag slipped off his shoulder and landed full force on my crotch. If I didn't need surgery before; I surely needed it now. What a way to go out!!

Get me to surgery fast!!!

6:30 p.m.

I found myself in a supine position. All I could see was a clock, what seemed to be a circular room, which resembled a space ship. Throughout this antiseptic area there were curtains—they were plain and colorless.

In my semi-conscious state, I could feel severe pain at the base of my back where it would meet the beginning of my rectum. It felt like a growth! It felt hot! It hurt! What the hell kind of surgery did I have?

19

Did I get the wrong doctor? Did I get the wrong surgery? What the hell is going on? I continued to do a reconnaissance of the area and spotted what could have been a human being. Was it a nurse? Was it an alien? What the hell were they doing? They kept moving in and out of the cubicles. I could see this creature writing something on what appeared to be a chart. But this creature kept moving in and out, writing, not writing, and so on. My managerial mind kept saying to me why can't they just do what they're supposed to do with one cubicle and be done with it.

As I looked again to where I thought the clock was; it appeared to have changed by an hour or so.

At the same time, I heard a voice in the room. "Please step aside. This is Romeo, I'm leaving now. Please step aside."

I was overwhelmed. As I looked over to track the voice; I saw what appeared to be a robot. He (it) appeared to display similar characteristics as found in $R_2 D_2$.

This was it!! This was truly a space-X!!X#! ship!! My body had been taken over by aliens! Holy Shit!! Did I die? Is this what it's like after death? Where the hell am I? Go to the light!! Where is the light? God, somebody help me!!

8:30 p.m.

My wife and son were permitted to see me in the recovery room. Another hour would have me in a room. Thank God, I'm still alive. I'm still on earth and not a part of it!!

20

CHAPTER 5

After-Care

9:30 p.m., Friday, July 24, 1998

Well, I finally made it to the ninth floor hallway. I was in a real live hospital bed, about to be placed into my room. I discovered that four bodies were required to move both me and the bed into these new confines. The room was large enough for two beds and two chairs. It included built-in wall lockers for personal belongings and a small bathroom.

My 70 some year old room-mate was moved out of the room while I was moved into the room.

I felt as though we were at an amusement park as it seemed I was in a "dodge em" car. My drivers left no stone unturned in finding anything that could be hit. It could also be compared to being a "bonus ball" in a pin-ball machine. Those flippers were indeed working over-time.

I was happy to learn through this process that I wasn't part of an alien spaceship. They really do have robots here at this hospital. They are primarily used to deliver supplies and medications.

Well, I'm finally settled, now for some rest. **WRONG!**

I received instructions that on an hourly basis I would have to attempt to cough. Additionally, I was given a plastic device with an attached plastic tube. I would be required to blow into this device at least 10 times in an hour period. The goal was to force the inner apparatus to move to a specific level. All of these efforts were supposed to reduce my risk of acquiring pneumonia. Not having been in a hospital as a patient for over 50 years, my goal was to get out fast. I coughed a lot and I blew into this plastic tube at least 20 times an hour.

Next, I would be equipped with some fashionable white nylon stockings. What are these? They were warm, electrified and pulsed. I learned these would help me in avoiding the development of blood clots, which might occur after surgery and cause some severe problems or complications.

My 70 some year old roommate was not happy. Why all this noise?

Now—maybe we could all get some rest. My wife spent the night with me, forced to try to sleep in a very uncomfortable chair.

But, who could sleep? We were visited hourly by someone testing this vital, testing that vital, taking some blood, and so on and so on.

7:00 a.m., Saturday, July 25, 1998

Welcome to the world of a teaching hospital. My eyes slowly opened as I sensed the presence of other human beings—many of them.

At the foot of my bed there appeared my surgeon, the student (who had taken my history) assigned to his service, the chief resident and almost a dozen medical students at various points in their budding medical careers. A discussion took place concerning my condition, procedures used within the past 24 hours and post-operative review of my situation.

Indeed, a Whipple Procedure had been accomplished. I would come to learn that part of my intestine was removed, 40 to 60% of my pancreas—gone, 40 to 50% of my stomach—gone, my entire gall-bladder—gone. Anything else?!?

Oh! I learned that I gained some things through out this procedure. I think I had a tube in almost every orifice they could find and then some.

The first one I can remember was the "NG" tube. I remember this one for several reasons, basically, because it was the first one to be removed and because it was probably the only one that would take my breath away upon removal.

The student assigned to Dr. Schroat advised me to take a deep breath. Before I knew it the "NG" tube came whipping out of my nose "faster than a speeding bullet." If my nose had been involved in a car crash, it clearly would have suffered from backlash. He had done a good job, but I felt like my navel had moved from its original position to the base of my esophagus.

Soon some more discussion of my condition ensued, while those attending got to gawk at my newly created incision. Seeming to be satisfied, the entourage departed. Little did I know or realize how often or how many would return.

8:00 a.m.

Next, I would be introduced to the shower. Please note I didn't say the bathroom had a shower. I was about to discover the "Brave New World" included an instant shower. Brought to your bed was a large clear plastic bag.

23

It included several white wash cloths and small white towels. In addition you were give two larger dry towels. The bag was very warm and the items inside were soapy and wet.

Welcome, instant bath/shower!! Bathe and dry yourself while in bed. Whatever works!!!

My wife was beginning to get a little agitated now (you must know she is not a morning person.) She set out on a mission to get me transferred to a private room—now!!

As the morning wore on, I would discover a plethora of new information that I would need to process. As promised by my physician/surgeon, I would be able to see the whites of my eyes and indeed a close inspection by my mirror proved him to be correct. Again, as promised, my skin would return to its natural color. Indeed, my skin no longer appeared jaundiced. In fact, my skin (by touch) seemed much softer and smoother, more than I can ever remember it being in the past.

The mirror provided me additional information. On the right hand side of my neck I had acquired approximately 6 to 10 tubes, all appeared to be color–coded. In fact, I looked as if I had acquired a number of dread locks suspended from my ear. I would come to learn that this was referred to as a "central line." Apparently, soon after you are under anesthetic, a great deal of action takes place including the insertion of a central line, from which blood was drawn for numerous tests.

I didn't need a mirror to conclude that I had an in dwelling catheter. I didn't need a mirror to figure out that a feeding tube had been inserted in my chest. I didn't need a mirror to determine that I had numerous "IV" lines inserted into my hand and arm. One may not say I was wired for sound, but I was certainly "tubed" for some type of action.

I didn't need a rocket scientist to tell me that I had developed (what would later be determined as) a bedsore at the base of my tail bone.

It is utterly amazing how quickly things can break down when you least expect. I definitely was in some pain from this development.

I didn't need a mirror to recognize that I had an incision down the center of my body as long as the eye could see. Keeping me together were approximately 40 plus staples.

I didn't need a commission from the United Nations on Hunger to tell me that I had not eaten since Thursday. I was hungry!!! I would soon find out that my diet would include ice chips and a flavored sponge on a stick that could be placed in ice-water for someone to give me a chance to suck on something. Is that all there is?

Keep coughing! Keep making that plastic machine move! Blow, Baby, Blow!

While my wife continued her crusade for another room, I would continue to be visited by medical students. "May I ask you some questions? May I see your incision? May I listen to your chest?" and so the day wore on.

I would soon meet the student, who had been specifically assigned to my case. He would come to be responsible in gathering most of my medical information. He seemed very young to me, but I would come to learn he was in his very early 30's and his wife was a nurse. He had reddish hair, a face full of freckles and if he wasn't cast for "Doogie Howser" he should have been.

He would diagnose the eruption at the base of my tailbone as a cyst, which would require surgery. My surgeon would later state this was a bed sore and the student didn't know what he was talking about.

As the day wore on, we continued to have blood drawn, blood sugars measured, the white nylons would be taken off and put back on, plugged in, plug taken out, "cough for me, blow into this device, please, thank you, get some rest now," and on and on. Then a new student would arrive, "I've just changed my rotation, may I ask you some questions? May I see your incision? May I listen to your heart-beat?" and on and on.

By mid-afternoon, my wife had achieved her objective. Be assured, a patient always needs to be an advocate or have one, who is persistent as the sun rising and setting.

My move began to take place. Another fun ride on the "dodge-ems" or as a bonus ball in the pin-ball machine. The hospital staff also provided for the installation of a "cross-bar" over the bed that I could grab on to in order to switch from side to side while I was lying in bed. This would help alleviate some of the severe burning pain at my tailbone due to the bedsore.

Of course, other wise, I was in little to no pain as I had another line (epidural) installed in my back. All I needed to do was push a button and I would receive an injection of pre-measured pain medication.

I told you I had tubes running in and out of me.

Keep coughing! Blow! Blow again! Harder! Blow again!!!

Throughout the rest of the day and through the night, I would be seen by someone on at least an hourly basis.

26

Students would arrive willy-nilly, but arrive they would. We would soon learn that the shorter the white coat— the lesser amount of knowledge. Conversely, the longer the coat—the more knowledge.

6:00 a.m., Sunday, July 26, 1998

"Good morning, how did you sleep last night?" I would reply, "I didn't. Someone woke me up every hour."

It would soon be time for an early morning visit by the Chief Resident and all his charges.

"Here they come!" At least, they now have more room to stand, be questioned, ask questions, take vitals, inspect incisions, and so on.

Next in line, once again, the microwaved instant shower.

I could smell breakfast trays—this iced sponge-on-a-stick and ice chips were beginning to get old.

My wife had spent the evening at the home of a friend's parents. She would return daily for an almost 12 hour vigil at my side.

Today my parents and mother-in-law would be driven by the same friends, who originally brought us to Pittsburgh for my initial exam. They were most gracious in transporting the senior citizen brigade to the hospital. I'm not sure anyone truly understood the gravity of our situation, but it was good to see them all and not have to worry about them attempting to navigate in the big city.

"Please cough! Breathe deeply and blow into the machine!" Oh, no, the white cotton electrified stockings again!!! I can't stand these pulsating gyrations!!

27

I was able to get out of bed and stand today. After I got all the tubes properly hung on my portable stand, I was able to move about the room.

I kept smelling food! Are these people trying to starve me or what? We received a number of phone calls and additional visitors this day so it was somewhat hectic. As the day wore on, I began to wear out. In retrospect, maybe that was good. "Push the button, just another shot for the pain!"

Sometime in the a.m., Monday, July 17, 1998

Oh! Oh! They're Back!!

Here comes the chief resident, here come the students, here comes the instant shower!!

A review of my condition would be conducted. Vitals would be taken, questions asked and answered, incision looked at, and so on.

The lead student (my boy, Doogie Howser) would come in to see me at 3 or 4 in the morning to see how I was doing and gather information that he would need for the 6 or 7 a.m. rounds.

I began to wonder if anyone slept.

Monday was somewhat of a "slow" day. However, I was able to get out of bed, saddle-up my tubes, hang them on my portable staff and begin to explore the halls.

While transversing and reconnoitering the area; I would meet fellow patients in the hall-way. All of us were at different levels of care and none of us were the same.

I remember specifically one encounter with a gentleman who stated he had his gall bladder removed. He asked me about my malady and I explained the "Whipple Procedure"

28

and the thought that I had pancreatic cancer. Amazingly he said nothing, but turned around and rushed down the hall and disappeared into his room. I was a little shocked by his reaction, but I would find similar reactions in the future. It seemed that once you said the "C" word, people would become standoffish. I don't know if they feared contamination or acquiring the disease themselves. In fact, I would later find some friends, who would purposely avoid shaking my hand. It seemed safer that way, I guess, at least to them.

I found a great deal of freedom and joy in my new found mobility. In fact, the Pittsburgh area was in the process of celebrating what was known as the "Ya Gotta Regatta," which is a summer festival on the 3 rivers surrounding the Pittsburgh area. This celebration included many vendors along the rivers, boat races, boat parades in the river, and decorated boats (similar to parade floats) for judging in various categories. I would spend the next few days attempting to convince individuals on the hospital staff that we re-allocate some beds, gurneys, wheel-chairs, "IV" poles, whatever and then we could decorate these and conduct our own regatta parade in the halls of the ninth floor.

Unfortunately, I got no takers and I think the feeling was that maybe I was pushing the pain button a little too often.

I will concede that I enjoyed being free and away from my bed as much as possible. This would allow me to avoid those damn white cotton stockings and unfortunately, my wife's uncanny ability to get her feet tangled in the various tubes lying on the floor by my bed. You don't want anyone to get mixed up with your catheter tubing and start to walk away from the side of your bed. You don't want anyone to

29

get lost in tubing to your central line or IV and start to leave your room.

I have to get out of here before her feet put me six feet under. But I love her; she's a jewel and a hell of an advocate.

Tuesday, July 28, 1998

We were beginning to make some strides today. The catheter was removed—what a relief that was!! The use of the electrified stockings had dramatically diminished.

Still no food, but the insertion of some nourishment through the feeding tube in my chest. This would be done in small amounts in short periods of time. It would also involve flushing the tubing system with water in between periods of feeding.

This was not my idea of a hamburger and fries, however, I still got to have ice chips and a cold wet sponge on a stick.

I continued my progress by getting out of bed as often as possible, saddling-up the tubes and going for a jaunt in the hallways of the ninth floor.

Everyday seemed to be a little better and I started judging progress by counting tube removal. One less tube—one less day!

Still no word on what the surgical team discovered when they got to do their internal exploration. My wife and I are becoming somewhat anesthetized to the results of any tests.

Wednesday, July 29, 1998

It's a good day—sort of...
No more white cotton stockings!
No more epidural tube for pain!!

No more "IV's" in my hand or arm for whatever reason!!!

Yes, still an instant shower!!

Yes, still a bedsore to deal with on a regular basis!

Yes, still the hourly blood draw, vitals, medical student visits, histories to be given, questions to be asked, and on and on.

This particular day, the Chief Resident stuck his head in the room mid-afternoon. My wife and I felt compelled to ask him what did they discover during surgery.

Surprisingly, he was quick to answer in a rather nonchalant, cavalier manner. "Oh, yeah, they got the tumor. Besides removal of a part of this or all of that, they took either 13 or 17 nodes during the procedure. I can't remember for sure but they found 7 of 13 or 3 of 17 or something like that, which had cancer."

Before we knew it, he had disappeared from the room and doorway. Before we knew it, my wife and I were in tears.

The only thing we had heard again was that frightening word, "Cancer!"

By some stroke of luck, I had a wonderful African-American head nurse, who had witnessed this encounter, as well as, two blubbering idiots.

She immediately sought out Dr. Shroat's associate, Dr. Kenneth Lee, who was doing follow-up care on my case since Dr. Shroat was now in Europe.

Within minutes, Dr. Lee was in my room and began to explain at great length and in miniscule detail what had actually transpired. He noted certain portions of my organs were cut away as they had been in direct contact or close enough to the pancreatic tumor to warrant such action.

31

In reference to involvement of lymph nodes, he stated that a total of 17 nodes were removed and explored. He believed a total of three showed positive for cancer. He explained the seriousness of my condition. Discussed again at great length treatment options which included surgery, chemotherapy, radiation, and so on. He told us about an experimental vaccine being tested at the Cancer Institute and that he believed I would be an appropriate candidate since this vaccine was only being used on pancreatic cancer patients. He would make a referral for us as soon as practical.

Our conversation ended and Dr. Lee continued on his rounds. His information and knowledge were helpful, but in the end, you remember one thing and one thing only—"you have cancer."

The rest of the day seemed to be uneventful, but this had been a day that seemed like an emotional roller coaster. I needed to sleep—and sleep I did!!

Thursday, July 30, 1998

Today began as other days with continuous tests, visits, vitals, instant hot shower and so on. At 3:00 a.m. I was visited by a new medical student. He stated he was on a new rotation and needed to discuss my condition, history, treatment, take my vitals, etc. "Did I mind if he did this?" "No, I don't mind it's only 3:00 a.m.!!"

I think I was getting a little short, stir-crazy and damn, I was hungry. It's been over a week since I have seen, let alone eaten real food.

By mid-morning, the Chief Resident returned. He asked if I was having a problem. He thought I seemed distant, detached, not my jovial self, preoccupied, and so on.

I explained to him that I was in deep thought and in the course of planning stages. I was attempting to devise a plan that would reap me personal edible rewards by hijacking the food cart that brought trays to my fellow patients.

Should I take a tray before it's delivered? Should I wait for someone's untouched/uneaten left overs? How could I do this and not be detected by hospital staff? Where and how could I hide the tray until I could get it returned?

I was pleased to hear him say that he thought he could get me some relief.

Lunch came and I waited and waited.

Alas, an angel of mercy appeared at my door and entered my room.

To my great delight, it had become Christmas in July.

On the tray, was a dish of shimmering lime jello. It was beautiful!! In another container, I found cranberry juice. Succulent, sweet, tart, wonderful, blissful cranberry juice! Oh, my God! This is heaven—this is truly Christmas, yet another container held hot tea. I've struck the mother-load!!

Eat slowly—relish every drop! Oh, how wonderful—I couldn't wait for dinner to come.

Dinner was almost as big of an event as lunch.

Jello—juice, hot tea—and chicken broth with crackers!!!

I've died and gone to heaven. I never thought I would obsess about food to this degree, but I think the longer I was confined the more "fixed" I became.

I started dealing with time based solely on meal delivery. I would listen for the elevator and the heated food cart. I would stretch to see if I could smell food on the floor.

Food, glorious food!!!

Friday, July 31, 1998

A very busy day that began with our usual burst of activity, visits, tests, questions, and so on.

Besides tube feeding, I was now on a soft diet. I think I hear the food cart. A scrambled egg, juice, tea.

By mid-morning, one of the medical students entered my room. He was of Middle Eastern descent and quite tall. In the past, he spoke very little, but I remember him copiously taking notes. I would later learn that he had a Ph.D. and would probably be a better researcher.

He told me his rotation was up and wanted to wish me well, but he was also here to remove the central line from my neck. He took all the appropriate precautions, (gloves, etc.) and set out to do his task.

Upon completion, he showed me what this thing actually looked like. It was not a pretty sight. I could only hope that I didn't have a cavern in my neck.

Later that afternoon, I was pleasantly surprised by a visit from my former pastor, Monsignor William "Max" Karg. He had spent approximately eight hours with my family and friends on the day of my surgery, but had to leave before I got to my room. I was so greatful to him for being there then and now. We spoke at some length.

Before he left he gave me a blessing and placed his hands on my head. I have never before, during, or since, felt such a burning heat that raced through my entire body. He prayed that whatever cancer or disease I might have would rid itself and leave my body.

34

I don't know if it did or didn't. But if it did—it happened that day and it happened that way!!!

Things were moving swiftly today. I think they were beginning to fear that I was going to eat them out of food within the next 24 hours.

Saturday, August 1, 1998

I called my wife at 10:00 a.m. at the home of a friend's parents, where she had been staying. Get ready—we're going home today. I should be released by 1 or 2 p.m.

"Doogie Howser" came into my room and asked me to lie down so he could remove the staples from my incision. He wished me well.

Other staff showed up; plans were being made for the visiting nurse and a local company to provide me with equipment and other food supplements for my feeding tube.

I think they wanted me out fast. They couldn't afford to keep feeding me.

My wife and I said our good-byes, discharge papers, instructions, etc. in hand.

We finally hit the road.

As we exited the city and got on to the inter-state, the radio was playing.

The song was being sung by Leann Rimes—"How Do I Live Without You?"

I looked at my confidante, chauffeur, advocate, lover, wife, friend and said: " How timely and prophetic can that be?"

We both began to cry and sob throughout the entire song. We didn't need to speak. We knew each other and what was in our hearts.

As we exited the inter-state, I was amazed at the feeling.
Was I in a scene from "Gulliver's Travels" or what?
Everything seemed so small! Was I a Lilliputian? It was
just bizarre.

As we arrived home, it was a flurry of activity. The
visiting nurse and the company representative with the
feeding tube equipment were there within two hours of our
arrival. Instructions completed and they were gone.

I was home—time to deal with reality!!!

CHAPTER 6

Chris's Ordeal

Sunday, August 2, 1998

Well, we're home—home, sweet, home! I would begin to spend a recuperative period on the "pit" in our den. I was required to lie at a certain angle in order for the feeding tube and process to work in an efficient manner.

By now, you can tell that we've had some "Daisy Days" some "Barbed-Wire Days" and some "Daisy/Barbed-Wire Days."

Most of today was spent dealing with phone calls and visitors. I continued to demonstrate an appetite (even though it was a soft diet), which was good. I needed to rebuild my system.

Since March of 1998, I had lost approximately 60 to 70 pounds. But there were more important things to be done now.

While in the hospital, we had received a number of phone calls from our primary care physician and Chris's surgeon in Pittsburgh. While checking on me and my post-operative condition; it was apparent (and rightly so) that both had a concern for my wife's health and well-being.

Bottom line was quite simple: if you don't have this surgery and the tumor is not removed, you will die.

Having seen her surgeon in July, the decision had already been made to have the actual surgery instead of a "laser" procedure. The "laser" procedure while effective could allow the tumor to return at a faster rate. The actual cutting away of the tumor would diminish that from happening with any great speed at all. The good news was that 95% of these tumors proved to be benign. We could only pray and hope.

The decision was made—surgery would take place on August 12, 1998.

Since I was unable to be there because of feeding tubes, and so on a plan was developed to get Chris to Allegheny with the help of family and friends.

Some friends would be assigned to stay with me during this period.

August 11, 1998

Chris left Meadville destined for the greater Pittsburgh. She would undergo pre-operative work-ups and surgery would take place the next day.

We kissed and she was gone and I would forever feel guilty that I was unable to be by her side as she was by mine.

In any event, later in the afternoon of August 12, we would get a call from friends as to her condition.

Apparently the surgery went well, the entire tumor was removed and initial testing found it to be benign.

Unfortunately, Chris was not doing very well and never does when anesthesia is involved.

She began to vomit, develop a leak of vital back fluids, was miserable and in the intensive care unit. When this information was conveyed to me over the phone, I began to cry and was unable to carry on any lengthy conversation.

She would get better!!!

She had to get better!!!

The surgery took place on a Wednesday and I was not able to speak to her until late Thursday. She was out of I.C.U. now, but still not out of the woods. Our conversation was very brief—"I miss you, I love you, get better, please!!!"

Late on Friday, we learned that Chris would be discharged on Saturday afternoon. She could come home to join the other walking wounded.

7:00 a.m. Saturday, August 15, 1998

This worked out well because I was scheduled to return to Pittsburgh for a post-operative CAT Scan.

Barb Iellimo, a dear friend both to Chris and I, was gracious enough to drive me to Pittsburgh.

39

I checked in with Out-Patient and moved to the Radiology Department. When my name was called I entered a small room and a lab technician gathered some information. At that point, a needle and tubing device were inserted into a vein in my hand.

I was given 4 cups of a liquid that looked similar to Kool-Aid and smelled like a watermelon. I was to drink so many cups in so many minutes and then a cup and a half in the next 40 minutes, saving a half cup to be consumed just before they performed my test.

One of the benefits in this whole process was that I learned since I had the "Whipple Procedure" I would no longer be required (or be able) to consume the magical white chalky substance.

Who said there isn't a benefit package here?

My name was called. I was escorted to a room, which had a device that looked like a half-eaten donut. Here I would be asked to lie down and the "donut-like device" would go back and forth scanning my lungs and all my other organs from top to bottom.

Hold your breath!!
Breathe!!

Hold your breath!!
Breathe!!

Now in the tubing in my hand an attachment had taken place. I was told at this point that they would now begin to allow iodine to flow into my body. I would feel some heat.

40

Oh, yeah!—Heat, indeed! It was hot and I could feel it throughout my body. Even my eye-balls felt HOT!!

The test itself was completed in less than a half-hour. The prep time was at least an hour and a half.

In any event, it was done. Now we could leave and back track north to Allegheny General and retrieve my wife from her ordeal.

As usual, we missed a turn. Honestly, I'm a better driver than navigator. I just never get where I'm supposed to go.

We were only off by one exit and so we got there at approximately 1:00 p.m. Our friend, Barb, would go up to Chris's room and get her belongings while I waited in the car. For some reason I was exhausted.

Eventually, Chris got discharged and was able to walk to the waiting car. To me, she looked beautiful!!

To you, she would look similar to a picture found in the *National Geographic Magazine.* While her face was somewhat swollen, she had various "stints" sticking out of her nose. The differences from pictures in the magazine were simple. She was white and not African. She wore more clothing. She was in Pittsburgh, not a village in Kenya.

Yes, she had sticks in her nose, but she was beautiful! She was my wife! She was alive! She was coming home! She was tumor free! She no longer had Cushing's Disease!!

The remainder of the day was spent in a rest mode. Here were two walking wounded, lying together on separate couches in the pit of our den.

The next few days were mostly uneventful and we muddled through the best we could.

Wednesday, August 19, 1998

Both Chris and I would return to the Pittsburgh area. She was required to see an ear, nose and throat specialist group, who were responsible for both inserting and removing the "stints" in her nasal passages. The removal took place without a hitch and it appeared that everything was as it should be.

Chris wanted to stop at a nearby mall before we returned home. I was captive and remained in the car. She needed to look for an out-fit, after all, our son was getting married in four weeks.

CHAPTER 7

Break Time—A Celebration

Aug. 16 through Sept. 19, 1998

The next few weeks were a whirlwind of activity. Going here—going there! Doing this—doing that! Appointment here—appointment there—appointments everywhere!!

I needed to get fitted for a tuxedo for the wedding. Chris was shopping for her third out-fit for the wedding. She had lost 30 pounds since her surgery. I had to return to Pittsburgh to see my surgeon for a post-operative visit—so did Chris. We both got permission to drink a little champagne at the wedding.

We spent one morning at the Regional Cancer Center, seeing a Dr. David D. Howell, Jr., who was in charge of radiation treatments, which would take place 40 miles north in Erie.

He spent a great deal of time talking to both Chris and me. Before this visit was over, we were all crying and hugging each other. He was a truly caring physician.

The plan was that I would go to Erie and get "marked out" for radiation treatments.

Later that afternoon, we received a phone call from Dr. Howell. He explained in great detail that he had had time to delve deeper into my files, medical history, and so on.

Based on his review, he came to believe that radiation treatments could be more harmful than helpful to me. Essentially and simplistically he stated, "Based upon your ulcerative colitis history and the reconfiguration of your organs as a result of the Whipple Procedure; radiation could possibly do more damage than good."

Decision—radiation therapy is not an option!!

For the past several years during the first week after Labor Day, a number of our friends would trek out to the Outer Banks of North Carolina. Generally, we would reserve a house on the ocean that would accommodate 12 to 16 people and this was done a year in advance. I insisted that we would meet our obligation—we were going. We needed an escape.

Normally, we would travel to one of our friend's house in Latrobe the night before we set out to North Carolina. We would do just that, but on this trip, the tube feeding would be an integral part of the trip.

We left Latrobe at 4:00 a.m. to meet other members of our group somewhere in Maryland for breakfast at 7:00 a.m. While in the van, I sat in the front seat with the feeding bag hung from the sun visor. The machine pump was good for 12 hours on a battery pack. Since I started the feeding late, I wouldn't be done until about noon. But we did get through the process and got to the Outer Banks.

44

We were greeted at our ocean-side house by some droppings in our driveway left by the famous wild horses. I took charge of feces removal and we were able to park as appropriate. I particularly enjoy this time of year for several reasons. I don't read a newspaper. I don't watch the evening news! I become one with the sun, the sea, the sky. There is nothing so splendid as a sunrise on the ocean, nothing as calming as hearing the waves kiss the beach, nothing as wonderful as the feeling of freedom when watching the dolphins roam the white caps. It's a wonderful escape!!!

While on this annual sojourn, I get to be the chief breakfast maker. You would die for my "Bailey's Irish Cream" French Toast or pancakes. I won't include the recipe here.

I think we had only one day of rain, a great deal of sun and fun!

Life was good! These were indeed some daisy days in spite of a feeding tube.

We returned home after the week and the return trip was uneventful. The following week would be spent in preparation for the wedding. I don't know how my wife did it, but she made dozens of cookies and so did other family members and friends.

The rehearsal and dinner following went off without a hitch. Just make sure I get there with check book in hand.

The plan was that my parents and mother-in-law would arrive by noon at our home. They were to be fully dressed as all of us had to be at the church by 1:00 p.m. for pictures.

My parents complied and were early as usual. However, my mother-in-law made it just in time, but was wearing regular street clothes.

She announced to my wife that she wanted a peanut butter and banana sandwich on some raisin bread she had brought with her. Chris told her (nicely) to make it herself since she was already dressed for the wedding.

My parents had situated themselves in the adjoining den and I was finishing lunch with a cup of pudding.

After I was done, I excused myself to the bathroom, which was adjacent to the kitchen and den. I needed to complete my tuxedo arrangement.

Much to my surprise, when I re-entered the kitchen I found my mother-in-law seated at the kitchen table with her treasured sandwich. For some reason, this 70 some year old decided to situate herself at the table in her panties, bra, and knee high stockings. Just what I wanted and needed to see today!!

I yelled upstairs to my wife to get downstairs. I was going outside to move the car out of the garage and into the driveway. I couldn't get out of the house fast enough.

Finally, the geriatric parade began to exit the house and enter the car. Time was becoming an issue. The last to arrive, of course, was my mother-in-law. She finally entered the back seat and I think half her dress got caught in the door. I stopped, she re-opened the door, closed again and we were off.

As we approached the church, the radio was blaring "I'm getting married in the morning" or some such song. As we parked the car; we could see the groom and the six ushers on the lawn east of the church. Beside them were two coolers; they were enjoying special libations.

Between them and my mother-in-law, I don't know what the church pastor was thinking.

In any event, we got there, got pictures taken and were ready for the big event. We got our parents seated and Chris and I returned to the front entrance to act as "greeters." At one point, one of the ushers slipped my wife a flask with some gin. This day—no matter what—was going to be a daisy day.

Parents of the bride and groom escorted their children separately down the aisle. Chris and I flanked our son. We got him down the aisle, hugged and kissed. Next came our future daughter-in-law.

The ceremony was beautiful and lasted approximately 40 minutes.

The bridal party exited and then came the parents of the bridal couple. As we exited, I wiped my brow as if to say, "Whew, that's over; we got it done." Strangely, family and friends began to stand and applaud loudly. I'm not sure who the applause was for, but life was good!!

The reception began shortly after the ceremony and ended after 9:00 p.m. I danced until I could dance no more. I had one drink during the entire reception, but had the bartender keep adding water and ice.

We would return home. Our parents would spend the night. I would get a late start on the feeding tube, but life was good. It had been a daisy day!!

CHAPTER 8

Therapies & Experimental Vaccines

August through Mid-November, 1998

As mentioned earlier, one of my surgeons (Dr. Kenneth Lee) had mentioned an experimental vaccine program being conducted at the Cancer Institute. He had referred my name to the individual in charge of this experiment, Dr. Ramesh Ramanathan.

We would come to Pittsburgh and first meet with the experimental program coordinator. She would explain in great detail what the testing involved, get release forms and other pertinent documents signed.

We would later meet Dr. Ramanathan, who provided us with additional information. In the simplest of terms, the vaccine is supposed to activate the immune system in order to protect the pancreas and adjacent organs.

The programs would last over a nine-week period and would entail, at a minimum, three vaccine injections spread out over the nine weeks.

Initially, I would be poked with a device similar to one used for tuberculosis testing and several vials of blood would be drawn. The goal was that some forms or bumps or lumps would show up on my inner forearm, which would support the notion that my immune system was working.

After the initial visit, we returned within several days to see if there was a positive reaction. I think 2 or 3 nurses and 2 doctors inspected my forearm, no one could find any reaction. Right now—you are not a candidate! I was crushed! I was not going to be qualified to participate in this test.

I think my reaction was so "devastated" that Dr. Ramanathan said we could try the test one more time. I got stuck again!

We returned several days later, success and luck and hope and faith were with us. Blood samples and skin bumps/lumps demonstrated an active immune system. We were a go!!

This vaccine required a special concoction of some type and was known as Muscin. I would be part of a second test group.

Each time that we returned to Pittsburgh, I would go to one location to have two vials of blood drawn. If the results were appropriate, I would be sent to the cancer out-patient treatment floor. There an additional 6 to 8 vials of blood were taken—some for testing and some for Dracula (I think). In any event, I would than receive an injection, which would later make my arm hurt and give me flu-like symptoms for about 24 hours.

In between the injections I would have to return to Pittsburgh at least twice within this nine-week period. At that time I would undergo skin biopsies being taken from the underside of my right forearm. There were at least two different sites on two different trips. Luckily, I would be able to go to my primary care physician to have the stitches removed from these biopsy sites.

In some instances we're talking about two trips a week to Pittsburgh. This would be a day long event. Almost two hours each way by car. Additionally, we would have blood work, get results, get more blood work, more results, wait for vaccine and a biopsy (skin removal) and so on.

The days were long and tiring, but my life was on the line!! I was willing to take any chance to beat the hand that had been dealt to me.

Remember, by the time we came home I was due to hitch up to my best buddy, the feeding tube, for my daily 12 hours of additional nourishment.

Throughout this process, Chris and I were shuffling schedules. In between all of this, we got in a week at the Outer Banks and our son's wedding, not to mention other events. I was beginning to need a personal secretary just to keep track of my medical appointments.

During this same period, a dear friend of ours (Frances Smith) had discussed with both Chris and I information regarding a support group for cancer patients. Fran, herself, had attended one in the past. We're we interested? Of course, as I said, I was going to do anything to get through this experience.

Our names were submitted and we were contacted. We accepted and Chris would attend as my support person.

I was amazed that at our first meeting there were almost 30 to 40 people. Some thin, some not so thin. Some having good hair days, bad hair days and no hair days. Some with breast cancer, ovarian cancer, brain tumor, prostate cancer, lymphoma, leukemia, me with pancreatic cancer, and so on. I told you I learned more medicine than I ever wanted to learn.

51

The program was conducted by Dr. Barry Bittman at the Mind and Body Center in Meadville, PA. A great deal of it was based on Dr. Bernie Siegel, a fellow pancreas buddy, who has survived over 15 years—an anomaly.

The program included support staff encompassing social workers, therapists, dieticians, nutritionists and so on. It discussed guided imagery, music, massage therapy, and many others over an approximate two month period.

Unfortunately, during these sessions, Chris spent a lot of time crying. I told her that I was convinced that when she had her surgery that the surgeon must have cut some tear ducts.

The program was positive and helpful. It got us through a very "barbed-wire" period.

We made some wonderful friends. We learned that none of us are alone. We learned that someone and everyone probably has or has had a heavier burden than you. We learned to bare our souls and for me I would also bear my skinny legs as I would always wear shorts no matter what the weather. I guess it became my "nom de plume."

We learned that some of us would return and some would or could not return. We learned to love by breaking down all the barriers. We laughed, we cried, we hugged, we shared, we cared, we died!!

We loved and oh! -- how we knew we had to laugh again and again!!

These were daisy days, daisy and barbed wire days and in a few instances, some barbed wire ones, too!

CHAPTER 9

A Diabetic Relapse

October, 1998

At the time of my surgery, I was advised that several things could happen after the surgery was completed relative to my diabetic condition. It might disappear (doubtful, but it could happen.) It could be controlled by mere diet and exercise. It could require oral medication, diet and exercise. It could become uncontrolled and require insulin injections, as well as, diet and exercise.

We were somewhat blessed after surgery because diet and exercise appeared to be working.

By mid-September, I had returned to real food and a regular diet. I had re-acquired my appetite. Life was good.

For some reason, however, my wife and I noticed that I continued to lose weight.

I continued my nightly tube feedings to supplement my food intake.

Remember my body was no longer the same as yours. I had lost parts of some organs and all of one. I was re-plumbed inside. My system needed support from a digestion level.

I was different, but life was good.

I would always tell my wife that after my surgery, the scar has now given me a "six-pack" look on my abdomen. Just a look!!!

Because of the incision, my navel is just a little to the right of center. I would insist that I kind of list to the right, like a ship taking on too much water on one side.

In any event, we continued to watch as weight continued to come down. We spoke to several doctors when appointments were kept, but could never really get any answers.

By the end of October, all hell broke loose. My blood sugar levels began to run wild and out of control. My levels were running between 300 and 400 on a regular basis.

During this same period, Chris was being followed up by an endocrinologist for her condition. Dr. Joseph Hines of Erie was working with her to monitor her condition.

October 29, 1998

I was watching Monday night football on this particular evening when my condition worsened. My diabetes was out of control. You know when your body just isn't working right.

Chris suggested that she contact Dr. Hines to see if he would take me on as a patient. She called him that evening and he was gracious enough to talk with her and agreed to see me.

The plan was established that we would drive to Erie the next morning to Hamot Medical Center, where I would be admitted for observation and treatment.

Diabetes is an insidious disease. It's frightening and devastating.

54

My father-in-law was a diabetic. I saw him lose a toe, a part of a foot, a part of his leg below the knee. I saw him die! His doctor said after his death that he had the organs of an 80 year old man—he was 55 when he died.

The disease had ravaged his body over the years and now my fear was that it was going to be my turn.

I would remain in the hospital from October 28th through October 31st.

After cancer, my second greatest fear was the need to take insulin by injection. There was no way that I was going to give myself shots.

WRONG!!!

It's amazing how fast you can learn to do something if you want to live.

I went through several sessions with a nurse instructing me on the mixing of Humalog and Humulin and doing it right. I learned to make injections in both my stomach and leg.

Frankly, I felt more comfortable giving myself injections in my upper leg. I was not quite sure how much of my stomach was left.

At any rate, a modicum of control returned and I would be discharged from the hospital on Halloween.

I could return home. Back to my couch. Back to my free standing "IV" stand. Back to my nightly feeding tube regimen. I was beginning to despise the sound of that machine running for 12 or more hours, but it was keeping me alive. It was a necessary support system. I began to call the "IV" pole/stand and equipment by name. It would now be referred to as "Herman" as I wanted it to become a "hermit" as quickly as possible. Only those who remember the singing group, "Herman's Hermits" will understand this illusion, but I was hoping my "Herman's" career would be shorter-lived than the actual singing group's.

After returning home, we began to settle into a routine. Testing blood two to four times a day. Insulin injections 4 to 5 times a day. Eating when I could, although, for some reason, my appetite was beginning to wane.

I continued to lose weight.

Chris and I would have several emotional discussions about my desire to continue to live. Many tears were shed. I was admonished that I needed to eat more.

The feeding tube could only do so much. You have to eat. You have to force yourself.

You have to want to live!!!

Thank God for Dr. Hines. Thank God that he was willing to take me on as a patient. Thank God for the ENDOCRINOLOGIST EXTRODINAIRE. He had now become another member of the team being formed. Only God knew what an important part he would play in this whole exercise of medical minutia.

Life was good even through the barbed-wire days!

CHAPTER 10

Introduction to the World of Oncology and Chemotherapy

In November, we would be introduced in great detail to the world of oncology.

We would meet Dr. Aiman Dhaghestani. He was from the Middle East, and was very well thought of within the medical community.

He would discuss at great length our situation. In fact, he was really the first physician that detailed how severe my diagnosis and prognosis were. He pulled no punches. He made no promises. He gave no guarantees.

All the things we were desperately seeking!!!

He, of course, like others before him (and after him) would complete a very thorough exam. I never knew that I had so many lymph nodes in so many places. I was beginning to feel like a Tell-a-Tubby, with finger-print indentations throughout my body.

The protocol for the treatments to follow was explained.

On each Monday morning, I would go to the local hospital for blood work. There would be a standing order for what needed to be tested.

Each following Tuesday morning, I would call a prescribed phone number to determine if I was a "go" for that afternoon to receive chemotherapy.

When I arrived on the chemotherapy floor, I would be weighed and my vitals would be taken. This would occur at approximately 1:00 P.M.

At that point, I would enter a room, which had approximately ten recliner chairs. Next to each chair was an "IV" pole and an extra chair for a visitor of the patient. The chairs were set up in a circle so that everyone was able to see everyone else. Strength in numbers? The ability to want to disconnect? At some point, you would be offered something to drink. Hopefully, it would help the medicine go down easier. RIGHT! Two or three nurses, aides and technicians were in and out of the room. At some point, Dr. Dhaghestani would appear and visit each patient. He was there and after seeing eight to ten patients, he would disappear.

My first encounter with blood work went off without a hitch and took place the first week of December. On Tuesday morning, I called and was cleared to come in at 1:00 p.m. for my first dose of Gemzar.

My wife felt compelled to join me for this first round. After passing through vitals, I sat in a recliner; I had psyched myself to get through this as quickly and as easily as possible.

My wife and I watched as personnel went around the room on a rotating basis to get people hooked-up for their very personal "trips and drips."

I noticed that the difficult part appeared to be getting a vein first of all and secondly, getting the needle works situated so that the therapy could begin. As it was explained to me at one point, essentially, there are two needles that somehow must work in concert with each other.

However, I'm no medical specialist or "techie" so just know that some people are just better at doing this part than others.

Always hope for good veins and a good "techie" so things run smoothly.

Well, it was my turn coming up after waiting in my recliner for about 40 minutes. The longer we waited, the more emotional Chris got. We needed the box of tissues for her again.

The nurse came up to us and asked our names again to insure who we were. I was ready!!

She was embarrassed and apologetic. She had just learned from supply that they did not have the needed chemotherapy item I was scheduled to receive. I would have to return tomorrow afternoon in order to receive my prescribed dosage.

Chris and I rode home—just a little upset---HOT!!!

I returned the next afternoon by myself as Chris had to work. Again I went through vitals and so on, but was ushered into an older private hospital room.

Unfortunately, I would see no fellow patients today since they did their thing yesterday.

Unfortunately, as well, my veins were not easy to find and the "techie" was not adept. It took three tries, but we finally made it.

The therapy itself would last approximately one hour. I returned home without event, but I was utterly amazed at how tired and exhausted I was. I think I slept from 2:30 to 6:00 p.m. that night. Just in time to try to eat and hook up to "Herman."

Several more treatments would occur and I would receive a one-week hiatus over Christmas.

I continued to be over whelmed at how tired I would get. It came to a point that my friend, Brian Kirberger, would drive me to and from the hospital.

I seemed to be getting weaker and more tired. I was given additional therapy to help with low blood counts—a natural reaction to chemotherapy, as I understand it.

It came to a point that I no longer had the strength or will to walk the driveway to get the mail.

I was losing weight, losing strength, losing the battle, losing the war!!

Christmas is coming—straighten up!!! You need to get some things done!!! You need to get through Thanksgiving first.

Parents, children, friends gathered for the annual fall event. We got through it. I was of little to no help to anyone.

This Thanksgiving was unlike any other that we had celebrated for the past 25 plus years.

I said a very personal grace and a word of thanks before our meal. It's hard to believe I even brought tears to my mother-in-law's eyes.

Many of our days were daisy and barbed wire days—But life was good!!!

CHAPTER 11

Christmas, 1998

It has been a wild roller coaster ride since July, "You have cancer." "You have a brain tumor!" "You have to have surgery!" "Radiation—yes, maybe, no!" "So, your son is getting married, when?" and on and on.

Prior to Christmas, of course, we celebrate Thanksgiving—and we, indeed, had much to give thanks for during this holiday season. Most important we were alive!!!

We spent Thanksgiving Day with dinner at home with family and close friends. The Friday after, my wife and our dear friend "J.D." would travel to the mall and begin the Christmas hustle and bustle. I was convinced that my wife was Bill Clinton's answer to a full and robust economy.

"J.D.'s" husband, Hank, would spend the day with me watching the annual football extravaganzas. We would annihilate making some turkey soup, but, nonetheless, would enjoy leftovers of the day.

The Saturday after Thanksgiving would be somewhat of a traumatic one for me. Both Chris and I had decided earlier that it was critical and necessary that we sell our apartment house that we had owned since 1972—our first home.

We had decided the quickest way to accomplish this was via an absolute auction. Three apartments had stood vacant since July, 1998. Utilities and other costs were mounting. Neither one of us was physically up to deal with this growing liability.

Strangely, it was interesting to note that over the past couple of years; we had encountered difficulties with a number of tenants. We had noticed that people just no longer felt compelled to honor their agreements and a lease to many was just meaningless. We had come to spend more time at the District Magistrate's office than we care to remember.

In fact, one former tenant still owes $1,200.00, but has since returned to Canada.

At any rate, the property was auctioned and unfortunately brought about $12,000.00 less than we had hoped. In any event, it was sold. The monkey would be off our back. Final closing would take place around January 10, 1999. The federal government would soon enjoy our capital gains—a lot more than we would.

Having said all that, Christmas was coming and in spite of weekly chemotherapy sessions, it truly was a wonderful time of the year.

I personally loved the holiday season. We would always have a live 6 to 8 foot Christmas tree. We would spend hours decorating our home, both inside and out.

The past couple of years we had two trees, one live and one artificial. The artificial would appear in the den to help celebrate and participate in Chris's collection of snowmen—I'm sure there are well over 300 of them now—no two alike.

I had always said that I would never have an artificial tree in the "great room" of our home. This year would be different—I didn't care. My heart was just not in it. I didn't want to decorate! I didn't want to celebrate!

Anyone who knows me would tell you that this is very much unlike me. Historically, it became a family tradition for our son to invite his friends over to watch and "hear" the annual event of getting the tree in the house, getting it set up right and decorated. This has been an event to behold. I remember one season when I dropped an axe and it fell gracefully onto the coffee table. The gouge lives on. Mostly, however, my son would want his friends to hear my Marine Corps-like Tirades. I do have to admit that they weren't pretty and believe me, after years in the Marine Corps, my language pattern had changed—dramatically and grammatically!! Oh, if Sister Veronica could only hear me now.

In any event, I had told Chris years prior that we would have an artificial tree over my dead body. Little did I know.

In the end, I told her to purchase an artificial tree. As I said, my heart and soul were just not in it. I continued to lose weight. I think I was down to about 140 pounds by this time. My strength and stamina were non-existent. Chemo was doing a real number on me. I no longer would retrieve the mail or take out the garbage. Each day I lost more of my appetite. My mouth became pasty inside. No matter how much I brushed, gargled, whatever, the result was the same. "Herman" continued to provide sustenance of sorts, but my bowel movements increased. I was getting weaker and weaker. Was I losing a battle or was the war all but over?

My friend, Brian, continued to get me to the hospital for tests and chemotherapy sessions. I would convince him to drive me to Erie on a Wednesday so that I could purchase some Christmas gifts for Chris—one being a diamond tennis bracelet.

Chris, our son and daughter-in-law and some friends, would set up and decorate the tree. I would only watch from the den as I saw them busily scurry about to get the job done that I used to love.

My wife (in her infinite wisdom) would go so far as to decorate "Herman." Before I knew it, the "IV" pole was decorated with artificial greens and lights. It was wired so that the lights would go on in concert with when the feeding tube was operational. To a degree, it would serve as a night-light as I continued to spend my entire days and nights on the couch in the den.

Christmas Eve at our home is a special event. Years ago we began a family tradition by having an open house. Initially, we did it because we wanted our son to be able to spend Christmas morning in his own bed and home. Our parents would come, we would have a special Christmas Eve dinner, we would attend a children's mass after dinner. Upon returning home we would have an open house for our friends. In the early years, this included friends and their children and would number about 20 to 25 people. Today, we have third generation children attending and we number anywhere from 60 to 75 participants, which usually depends on weather. It's a wonderful time of the year and Chris and I love to entertain with food, fun, libation, friendship and love.

This Christmas Eve would be greatly different. I would try to eat some dinner. We would not attend church services. I would be hooked up to "Herman". I would not be able to entertain and take care of the drinking needs of our guests.

At one point in the evening, I would have to excuse myself and find solace in one of the bedrooms. My diabetes had kicked in full force—I was having a reaction. I was sweating, but I was cold. I needed some sugar and drank some orange juice. It was not a good night!!! I was of no help to anyone and I knew it.

After our guests left, we would exchange gifts between parents, ourselves and children. We completed what (on this night) I considered a task.

I would hook myself up to "Herman" for a relatively restless night. I didn't feel well and I knew it. Weaker, whinier, short-tempered, tired (always tired) and afraid, very much afraid!!!

We would spend additional time with Chris's relatives over the next week and a half, both at our home and her cousin's.

Again, I would have to excuse myself to the solitude and sanctity of our bedroom. My blood sugars were going haywire.

We would spend New Year's Day at one of Chris's cousin's home. I ate some, but not much. Again, a pasty feeling in my mouth would reduce my appetite, my willingness to eat or drink. The men would gather, eat, drink and watch football in the den. The women would spend time in the dining room. I could hear Chris talking about and showing off her tennis bracelet. Then there were tears and crying and I would yell out, "knock it off!" She did. I'm glad I got her the bracelet. It only expressed in the most minute detail what and how I truly felt.

My hope was that there would be more Christmases and more New Years to celebrate.

Only time would tell!!!

CHAPTER 12

A Downhill Slide

Slowly, softly, sadly, slipping away.

The new year was not looking too good for me. I continued to lose weight. I continued to lose my appetite. I continued to lose my strength. I continued to lose my will.

My body weight was now between 130 and 140 pounds. As each day passed, I seemed to be weaker. It was more difficult and more time consuming to walk. Since I had to go up two flights of stairs to the bathroom in order to get a shower; I was engaging in that task later and later each day. I began to lose interest in almost everything. "Herman" continued to provide the continuous whining noise that seemed to keep me alive. Little did I know or realize that it was, indeed, "Herman," who was providing the basic nourishment I would need to survive.

The first two weeks of January of the new year were filled with blood tests and subsequent chemotherapy sessions. If my memory serves me, one of those treatments required that I be moved to a private room since I was running a low-grade temperature.

I would also learn throughout this process that there were control valves that would and could regulate the flow of the medication during the chemo session.

I would learn that the faster the drip would mean the sooner your session would end. It would also provide a great burning sensation at the location where the needle was placed. You could control this indirectly by speaking to the nurse or technician that was conducting your session.

Each was gracious and would turn the valve up or down, depending on what your wishes were.

Again, I was blessed to have Brian as a friend. A retired school teacher; he was able to take the time to get me to the hospital for both my tests and treatments. Unfortunately, my condition was making it more difficult to get up into his high step truck, but we managed.

In my mind, my diseases (all of them) and my battles with them were beginning to isolate me. I was becoming an island, a man without a country. The weaker I became in body strength; the weaker I became in my will to fight and struggle.

Thank God for my wife. She would always say the right thing at the right time. She would always be able to bring me back to center.

However, this time I wasn't sure about anything. I began to believe this was bigger than any of us ever imagined. I didn't want to "exit—stage right," no, not just yet—not without a fight.

If being in the Marine Corps for four years taught me anything, it taught me this—You can survive anything! You can win—but you must fight with a gusto, zeal and fervor that no one can achieve for you, but you yourself.

The Marines' motto of Semper Fidelis (Always Faithful) not only applied to the unit, to the team, to the objective; but it also applied to one's self. I would have to be faithful to myself.

By no means do I consider myself a religious person, but I do think of myself as a faithful one—that is, full of faith. As things were going, I didn't have many other choices and I didn't like the remaining option.

Both Chris and I were blessed with many family and friends who supported us through these six months.

Between the two of us, we received over 500 cards, notes and letters. I can't begin to count the gifts, hospital and home visits, telephone calls and so on.

I know that our names have appeared in at least four or more prayer lines in Erie, Meadville, Pittsburgh, Virginia, and God only knows where else.

Countless numbers of people were praying for us—Christian, Jew, Muslin, Hindu. There were people we would never come to know, never learn their names, their positions in life and so on.

It was amazing that you could feel a power, a strength, a pulling. No words can describe this feeling, but it was truly there just like the heat when Monsignor "Max" laid his hands on my head.

The sense was that something was happening. But what? Was it a false hope? Was it faith? Were the prayers working? I don't know. Something was. All I know was that God wasn't done with me yet—there's a plan here somewhere!

CHAPTER 13

On Death and Dying

January 18, 1999

Martin Luther King's Birthday Observance

I had just hung up on "Herman" in the early morning and was trying to get a shower. This, of course, was Monday and as part of my normal routine I would have to get to the local hospital and have some blood drawn in order to see if I was still a "GO" for chemotherapy on Tuesday afternoon. The morning was pretty much uneventful, but Sunday in the late afternoon was more than memorable for me, at least, as I look back on it now.

That late Sunday afternoon I decided to go upstairs to our bedroom and watch the Pittsburgh Steelers attempt to play football. I took with me a can of Dr. Pepper, I can't remember if it was diet or not.

I watched the game for some time while sipping away. Suddenly, I felt the most horrific pain in my stomach area. I had never ever in my life felt such a pain. Frankly, it brought me to my knees and I was in tears.

Chris was downstairs (thank God) and saw none of this. I went to the bathroom to seek some insured privacy. I was writhing in pain. I made every promise to God that I could think of at the time. I will never drink another Dr. Pepper again, just make this pain go away or let me die. Please, please, I beg of you just let this pain go away.

And God answered me; the pain subsided to the point where I was able to return to the bedroom. Unfortunately, the pain returned--unfortunately, stronger than the first experience. I wasn't sure if it was Dr. Pepper or the poor playing of the Steelers that was causing this pain. To be honest, I don't even remember who won the game.

I would return to my knees in the bathroom and pray for relief. God was good and relief came. The day was a mix of daisies and barbed wire.

I spent somewhat of a restless night concerned about this unknown pain, both ascending and descending in strength. Time to hitch up to "Herman:" morning would come.

As I mentioned, it was Martin Luther King's birthday observance. Chris was off of work that day but planned to keep the "Bill Clinton economy" going full speed ahead by traveling to the mall. She was and is very patriotic. She asked if I minded since I hadn't seemed too chipper at dinner Sunday evening. I replied in the negative.

As the day wore on, I had had my shower, gone to the hospital and returned after having blood drawn.

I had tried to eat some breakfast, took my pills, took my insulin and quietly sat on the couch.

While the pain of Sunday night had subsided dramatically; I was still whipped by the whole event. I never wanted to experience that type of pain ever again.

I continued to feel that somehow I was slipping away from all that was real. I was becoming more and more isolated. The more I tried to get better; the more difficult it would get. Was I really losing the battle and the war?

Prior to all of these past six months, I was always in fear of my death and dying. Over the past few months, I had come to some different realizations.

I really wasn't afraid of death and dying. I had come to learn that they were one-time events. They could hurt for the moment, but I would never have to relive them again.

What I really learned that I was afraid of was not living. Living was an on-going event. It was more than a daily activity. My fear really surrounded all the things I would miss and not be able to be a participant. The parties, the get-togethers, the trips to the Outer Banks, the quiet conversations with my closest and dearest friend—my wife, and so many other wonderful human things.

Lunchtime would come and go. I attempted to eat some soup. I got about half of the broth down. Tried to drink some fluids. Everything was tasteless.

Attempted to go to the bathroom a number of times but nothing seemed to be functioning. I felt as if I had the testicles of a flea. I was beginning to disappear before my very eyes.

I now had the body of what I would call an "Aushwitz victim." I was down to 130 pounds. In six months I had lost nearly 90 pounds. I think I was dying.

I didn't even attempt to have dinner or hook up to "Herman." I was in trouble—real trouble!!!

Chris returned from her shopping marathon around 9:00 p.m. that evening. When she came in the house, I think she had a sense that our lives were about to change again.

I told her we needed to go to the hospital. I didn't know why, but we had to get there and get there soon. She called our son, who came the five miles to our home as soon as he and the weather would allow him. It was mid-January and a snow storm was brewing.

Scott had to help me from the den and get me to the car in the garage. By this point, I was unable to walk unless someone assisted me. I think it had something to do with my dehydrated state.

In any event, Chris would drive me to the hospital and Scott would follow in his vehicle.

We got to the emergency room before 10:00 p.m. and I was taken in by wheelchair.

Efforts were made to get an "IV" running and after several attempts, someone found a viable vein. I would also be given oxygen.

At some point, I was moved from an examining room down the hall to x-ray. I could feel the cold stainless steel table against the bones in my back. We would discover that I had suffered a double perforation of the bowel.

I was in real trouble! I was truly near death's door. No one at the local hospital wanted to touch this.

A call was made to Pittsburgh in an effort to contact Dr. Schroat. He was unavailable, but Dr. Kenneth Lee was covering. The plan was made to transport me to Presbyterian Hospital in Pittsburgh.

Initially, the plan was to "life-flight" me via helicopter. This was later ruled out because the weather had gotten so bad because of the snow storm that no flights were getting clearance. The second plan quickly took shape and I would be transported by the local ambulance company. My wife would ride up front with one EMT as the driver. The second EMT and a nurse from the hospital would ride with me in the back.

I needed some more work done on getting some fluids and the nurse's were having no luck. The EMT did it the first time without a hitch.

At approximately midnight, we would leave the local hospital for Pittsburgh. Our son would follow in our car.

As we left the emergency room parking lot, the EMT and I had been strapped into position.

Unfortunately, the hospital nurse (who, as I remember, was short and stout like a teapot, was not in position.) She was standing above and to the left of me as the driver hit a pothole two blocks from the hospital. The nurse lost her balance and as a result, fell on top of me full force. She used both her hands to try to brace herself, but landed directly on my stomach.

If I wasn't dying then, I wanted to be dying now. She was very apologetic, but I think I heard someone say, "Come to the light!"

The further south we drove, the less snow we encountered. Approximately twenty-five miles from Pittsburgh, the ambulance made an unscheduled stop on Interstate 79.

Chris thought that I had died since no one told her anything about stopping or gave her any reason.

As it turned out, the stop was needed to test my vitals to determine how much (if any) morphine I could be given.

At this point, Chris tells me my blood pressure was 60 over 30. She wasn't sure of the pulse rate, but she knew it was low.

I was well on my way to the **LIGHT!!**

At approximately 2:00 a.m., under the bright lights of the emergency entrance at Presbyterian Hospital, we arrived.

The nurse and EMT's wished us well. I was wheeled into and transferred to an exam table in the emergency room. It seemed as if everyone was walking in slow motion.

Was I back on the local space ship?!

CHAPTER 14

The Big City Revisited

Tuesday, 3:00 a.m.
January 19, 1999

After watching what seemed to be hundreds of people walking in slow motion, I fell into a heavy sleep.

I would come to learn that I would undergo 6 to 7 hours of surgery for a double bowel perforation.

Coupled with this of course, were some additional attending complications. Namely, besides your ulcerative colitis, diabetes and pancreatic cancer, you not only have bowel perforations—but, you also have peritonitis.

In the simplest of laymen's terms, you have an accompanying massive infection.

Thankfully, Dr. Lee would perform the surgery.

Remembering back to the previous Sunday and the severe abdominal pains while drinking Dr. Pepper would now make a lot more sense. If it didn't make sense, at least now I could explain the pain.

The surgery began at approximately 3:00 a.m. on Tuesday morning and would last until 9 or 10:00 a.m.

These folks had some heavy-duty work to accomplish during this procedure. Not only did they have to clean me out and irrigate my entire system, but provide antibiotics to help fight off and destroy any infections.

I wasn't as lucky this time as I was when I underwent the "Whipple Procedure."

This time I would require approximately 4 pints of blood and volumes of fluids to hydrate my system. As I understand it NOW, I was admitted in a state of being dehydrated. This action was required to get me back to some level of normalcy.

The surgery was completed within the described time frames, but wasn't done yet. I required so many fluids and antibiotics that the surgical team was unable to reclose the original incision.

In other words, I was lying there on the table with a gaping open wound. I was transferred to the intensive care unit where I would begin to spend a four to five day stay.

At this time, I had no idea who I was or where I was, nor did I necessarily care.

I was in and out of consciousness—mostly out, at least as much as I can recall.

CHAPTER 15

Where Am I?

As I moved back and forth from consciousness to unconsciousness, I began to notice that this hospital visit was unlike my first experience.

No one came into my room and instructed me to blow into a plastic device in order to insure that I didn't get pneumonia and that I would have clear lungs.

They didn't have to provide those instructions.

I was on a respirator.

I didn't know and I didn't care.

I remember how thirsty and hungry I was after my surgery in July.

This trip—I didn't know and I didn't care.

I was on a plethora of drugs during this period. In retrospect, I think too many.

Of course, there were the necessary IV fluids and antibiotics. And too, there was the wonderful and not so wonderful morphine.

I would lay in a supine position for four to five days. During this same period, I would have an open wound. I could feel its openness. It felt as if it was a breathing thing. It was filled with fluid and gauze dressings. From time to time, it would feel as if I was being moved from side to side. During that same event, it would feel as if fluids were running out and down the side of my body.

Where, in God's name was I, and what was I doing here? I started to feel like a reading from Genesis about God and the act of creation. All I could think of was, "...night fell and morning followed. Night fell and morning followed," and on and on. But I never heard God say, "...it was good..."

I can remember people, (very close people,) like my wife, son, daughter-in-law and J.D. (Joy Dunbar) coming in and out of the picture within my mind. I can remember seeing them. I can remember hearing them. "Do you know where you are?" "Do you know who I am?" "Do you know what day it is?" "Do you know what time it is?" "Is it day time or night time?"

I remember the questions—I don't recall the answers. Night and day were the same to me. I remember no sun, no moon. I remember no light, no dark. Days would rush into night and vice versa.

Who was I??

Where was I??

I didn't know!! I didn't care!!

Please, please just release me and let me off this space ship. I no longer want to be a part of this laboratory test. Please, please just let me get off.

As time went on, I became more aware of my surroundings. I would later tell my wife that one of the nurses snuck me an orange Popsicle. No nurse ever gave me a Popsicle during my intensive care visit.

I remember the doctor coming in and stating that I would have to return to surgery as they would have to attempt to put me back together again both on the inside and out. Apparently, because of being hydrated, they couldn't

80

achieve that during this first go around. It was critical that I remain as clean and sterile as possible. Infection could be very critical and harmful to my well being.

I remember the day or night before my next surgery. There was a new nurse that was on the scene. This was a male nurse that I had never seen before and I was concerned. This individual actually frightened me merely by his looks. He sported a moustache. Not just any moustache, but one that was modeled after the handlebar moustache of older days.

This man frightened me. He just had this strange look about him and he reminded me of the character, "Simon-Bar-Sinister." He just gave me the creeps!!!

I guess night time came and before I knew it something was happening to me. I believe some device was inserted in my rectum. Later, I would have a bowel movement while lying in bed or whatever I was lying on. I was distraught!! I could hear people laughing. I could see this male nurse laughing. I was being rolled from side to side.

Were these aliens? Were they performing some bizarre exams or tests? Why were they laughing at me? Had someone raped me? Why was I having this discharge?

What the hell is going on? What are these people doing to me? What are they doing to my body?

I felt violated!! I felt strange!! I felt lost!! I felt alone!!

Was I dreaming? Was this some kind of nightmare?

Night fell and morning followed!!!

Before I knew it I was on a gurney with two young orderlies wheeling me down a myriad of corridors and hallways. I had never been here. It was freezing and I was freezing. The overhead lights were strange and foreign to me. I had never seen anything like them before.

I was indeed on a space ship and was about to undergo whatever the aliens deemed appropriate.

I arrived in what I would call a holding area and I could see other gurneys or carts lined up against the outer walls.

I made up my mind at that point that these aliens weren't going to take me without a fight. I was informed that I would be going into surgery. It was supposedly 7:00 a.m. I advised whoever was there and whoever was listening that no one was taking me anywhere.

I wanted to see my wife and if I was truly having surgery, I wanted to see my surgeon, Dr. Lee.

I was asked by a number of individuals if I knew who they were and if I remembered talking to them. I replied in the negative and that they all looked the same to me. No one was moving me anywhere—anytime!!!

As time went on, numerous people would come up to the side of my gurney and attempt to speak to me. When I looked at them, they appeared to look like someone you would see looking through a keyhole in a door way. Your face and body would appear to be not in human form, unreal, strange, bizarre, alien.

Finally, my wife appeared on the scene. Thank God. Someone real and someone I could trust. She would save me!! She would get me off this space ship!!! She would get me home safe and sound and secure!!!

I explained my dilemma to her. I explained to her about the male nurse, the suspected rape, the "Simon-Bar-Sinister" look-alike moustache. I discussed at length my rectal discharge and the embarrassment, laughter and so on. I pulled back the sheet covering my body and said look at this. I was lying in a puddle of a semi-bowel movement.

82

I told her Dr. Lee said it was imperative that I be clean and sterile before they do this surgery and look at me. I told her she had to get him here to clean me up.

She did her best to settle me down. Informed me that no doctor (including Dr. Lee) would be cleaning me up, but someone would before the surgery took place. I told her about the aliens and the space ship.

Finally, I told her if I'm right, I won't be back. I insisted that she take my wedding band so that when I don't come back, she'll know I was right. She finally got me quieted down to the point that she could leave and I could be taken to surgery. They were now almost two hours behind schedule.

Needless to say, I was hallucinating! I was delusional! I was psychotic!!

In a discussion held with my wife, the doctor could only explain it in two ways. My condition was either caused by drugs, in particular, the morphine, or something that is referred to as intensive care psychosis. This being a reaction to the location, type of care, length of stay and so on.

In any event, he told her had she not settled me down; the plan was not to take me into surgery in that condition.

As the day wore on the second surgery took place and lasted approximately three hours.

While this surgery was not as eventful as the previous two, one could only say that the pre-surgery activities of this one were no match for any of the others. I can only imagine what was going through the minds of these medical students.

They certainly got their money's worth this semester and I didn't even try to make it happen. I do know this, however, keep me away from morphine. Keep me away from ICU's! Keep me away from hospitals for a long, long time and whatever you do, keep me away from any space ships in the area!

After this surgery, I think I spent another two days in the intensive care unit. From there I was transferred back to my old floor at Presbyterian Hospital.

My wife had made arrangements this time in advance to insure that I would be transferred to a private room.

And private—it was. Unfortunately, this room had previously been a walk-in closet of sorts for all the linens on the post surgical floor. I would last here about three days before being transferred to another private room.

I found the linen closet experience interesting because in order to get to the other side of my bed, the medical staff would have to physically move the bed to the other side of the room. This should give you some idea as to the smallness of the room.

An operation report reveals that this last surgery took place as a result of the previous surgery, "Because of the swelling and edema of his abdominal organs and abdominal wall at the conclusion of the operative procedure, it was not possible to close his abdomen and his abdomen was packed open at that time. He returns now for irrigation of his abdomen and possible closure of his abdominal incision. The indications for the procedure, alternatives and potential risks which include but are not limited to bleeding, infection, the inability to close his abdomen, the possible need to use prosthetic material to do so, the possibility that his anastomoses will not be healed and will require revision in some fashion , as well as cardiac, pulmonary,

84

neurologic, renal and hepatic complications were discussed with the patient and his wife, who understand and agree to the planned procedure."

We sure did agree!! We were walking a medial tight-rope and we knew it.

After performing the operative procedure, "...we then packed the wound with Kerlix gauze, moistened with anti-biotic containing saline. The procedure was performed without complication and tolerated well by the patient... in stable satisfactory condition."

The bottom line to all of this was that they were able to sew everything up on the inside that was necessary. The outside would remain open and be allowed to heal from the inside out and eventually close on its own.

I would have an open wound, which would require a change in dressings twice a day for the next several months.

Back to the private room. In short order even the medical staff were dismayed with the arrangements and within three days, I was moved to a more spacious room with a half a bath.

It was now nine days since I was initially admitted to the hospital. I had nothing to eat or drink except IV solutions and ok, yes, now I was back on the feeding tube. Surgery had removed the old device and inserted a new one.

I can only think this was done because of a fear of possible infection with the old device.

In any event, a new twist to the situation occurred. I now began to have chronic diarrhea. Was it from the tube feedings? Was it from the actual product being used in the tube feedings? Was it a result of the surgery? Was it something else? 85

In any event it wasn't pretty!!! I continued to be poked and prodded as before. My blood sugars were under control with insulin injections. Blood sugar levels were tested very two hours. It got to a point where I just told the technician to squeeze my finger and something would come out without being pricked again.

I have to admit early on that while I was in the first private room, Chris gave me back my wedding band. I was glad she did, but I was more glad that the delusions and hallucinations had gone away.

As far as the diarrhea went, medication was ordered and it seemed to slow the problem, but not eliminate it. The dietician then ordered a different brand of supplement to be used in the feeding. It too helped slow the problem, but not eliminate it.

One has to remember now that I had lost over 90 pounds, now weighing in at 130 soaking wet. In addition, I had lost almost 75% of my muscle mass. I was unable to get out of bed on my own! I was unable to stand alone! I was unable to walk! I was one flaming mess!!! Is there any wonder why I ended up in adult diapers?! How embarrassing is that?

As before, the medical staff on the floor was most gracious and supportive. I can only recall one individual (a beautiful, blonde, blue-eyed young lady,) who had just chosen the wrong profession.

I would be visited by physical and occupational therapists on a daily basis. They were working feverishly to get me back to a higher level of functionality. I appeared to have been taken out of an Aushwitz or more recently, Serbian death camp. I was not a pretty sight.

I still got the good old instant showers. I think it would take me an hour to get through the process. Shaving? Brushing of teeth? Washing of hair? I didn't know—I didn't care. I just wanted out of here. Of course, we continued with daily student visits, a new chief resident, but we've already been there. So, you know the drill.

Still no food. I didn't care. I hadn't even considered hijacking the food cart when it came to feeding.

Finally, on one day, the diarrhea problem seemed to be under some control and someone ordered that I start on solids with the evening meal.

I was served that night with stuffed manicotti shells and my vegetable was spinach. I don't remember anything else. However, this meal was served about ten minutes before the chief resident and medical students showed up.

My wife had tasted it and said it was awful. She asked the chief resident if he would eat this and he replied they had the same food. Chris was incongruous how anyone having my surgery and subsequent problems would be expected to eat this.

In any event, thank God the nursing staff saw this fiasco, got me some mashed potatoes, jello, chicken broth and apple sauce to work around.

It was good, but a slow process. It was almost like learning to eat again. I was shaky. Was it my post surgical weakness? Was it low blood sugars? Was it just weakness due to weight and muscle mass loss?

It really didn't matter. It was going to be a longer road home. I continue to progress slowly and regain some strength. I was now able to get out of bed, but still required assistance. I could walk with the use of a walker, but only about 150 feet. I would then need to sit and rest so that I could make the return trip to my bed.

There was no racing the hallways with IV poles as there had been in the past. There was no talk of "Ya Gotta Regatta" and building floats for an in-house hallway parade. It was different this time. I was different this time. Life was not the same, nor would it ever be the same again.

I was changed and my life had changed and there were many changes yet to come.

As time progressed, so did I. While I had visitors during this period, they were few and far between. After all, it was winter—the middle of winter and most (if not all) our family and friends were well north in the "tundra." Secondly, I know I was not and would not be the best company.

I still displayed some evidence of chronic diarrhea, but this had subsided. I was eating more. I was re-gaining some level of strength. I would have both occupational and physical therapy evaluations.

It was determined that I could not return home, but would require 3 to 4 weeks in a rehabilitation unit to bring me back to a level of acceptable functionality and mobility.

February 5, 1999

I would be discharged in the afternoon from Presbyterian Hospital and transferred via ambulance to Health-South Rehab Hospital of Erie. I would return in a week to see Dr. Lee for a post-operative review of my condition.

It was time to move on.

Some days were daisies, some were barbed wire and some were days of daisies and barbed wire!!!

CHAPTER 16

Learning to Walk Again

Afternoon, Friday, February 5, 1999

I would arrive at Health South in Erie sometime in the late afternoon. My friend and advocate had already made arrangements for my room.

The ambulance trip was mostly uneventful and I had said my fond farewells to the hospital staff as my wife supplied all three shifts with pastries from a local bakeshop.

I had a back-end view of every pothole on Interstate 79 as we drove the nearly three-hour trip to Erie. I am convinced that (1) orange and white barrels are really state flowers and (2) ambulances have absolutely no insulation or sufficient level shock absorbers to help defer some of the jolt and shock of an uneven road. I truly can see why and how long-haul truck drivers could give Pennsylvania's highways such low grades. And think just how high up off the ground they get to sit.

As I arrived, the two EMTs proceeded to get me through halls and elevators faster than I could ask if we had arrived at the mother ship.

I was ushered into my room and transferred to my bed. There was an assortment of medical staff waiting to attend to my needs. Chris was scheduled to arrive later that evening.

My paper work and orders were given to those in charge and the process of getting me acclimated to my new surroundings began with barely a breath to spare. These folks were certainly efficient or they all had Friday night dates and wanted an early start to their weekends. I obliged as much as I could.

I was seen by the social worker, who collected necessary data and history. While she was there, I, unfortunately had a severe abdominal pain and an associated diarrhea event. I think when she saw me in such pain that all the blood rushed from her face. She was as white as my sheets. She informed me she would get the nurse and we could finish our interview at a later date.

Before too long, I was hooked up to this facility's version of my "Herman." Some things just never change. I was brought some type of food, but I don't remember what it was.

Vitals were taken, blood sugars, insulin administered. Chris would arrive later after completing numerous errands. To this day, I don't know how she kept up and kept going and kept it going!! She is truly a marvel and epitomizes the intent in our marriage vows of "in sickness and in health." I was certainly giving her a run for her money in that area. In fact, I think I was beginning to develop an undesired expertise.

It was nice to be somewhere else. It was nice to be closer to home, family and friends. It was nice to get some rest.

Oops! Forgot to check your blood sugar. Forgot to get your insulin. Forgot to change the dressing on your open wound.

A vast number of people wanted to see that wound so that they knew what they were dealing with on a daily basis. I was more than willing and happy to oblige.

Now let's settle down for some rest.

Don't forget the 3:00 a.m. insulin injection after your blood sugar has been tested.

"Did you sleep well last night?"

Saturday, February 6, 1999

Happy Birthday to me! Happy Birthday to me!! Happy Birthday dear meee! and so on.

Hard to believe I just became 55. It seems more like 65 today. Where have the days gone? Where have the weeks, the months gone?

Today and tomorrow would be somewhat slow days as most of the therapists were off for the weekend. While there was some activity with some patients, it was very limited.

I would be seen today by Dr. Robert Schwartz of Erie as I was referred to him by the Rehab Hospital's Director, Dr. Conrado Toledano.

He was concerned with my continued chronic diarrhea and wanted a consult.

Dr. Schwartz was an amicable guy. Very smart and intuitive, very comprehensive and interested. In the end, (no pun intended,) he felt that my problem could stem from multiple factors. Namely, the chronic diarrhea could be caused by:

91

1. Pancreatic insufficiency due to the Whipple Procedure.
2. The type of antibiotics I was taking.
3. The history of ulcerative colitis.
4. The tube feedings, or
5. The Gemzar chemotherapy, which causes diarrhea in almost 20% of patients receiving that treatment.

Dr. Schwartz would place me on additional medications and a lactose-free diet. Additional studies and tests would be done as a follow-up measure.

Interestingly and thankfully within the week, some normalcy began to return to my bowel movements. One incident occurred with blood in my stool, but close watch provided no other incidents. It could have just been strain.

Later that evening, there must have been a dozen or more visitors in my room to celebrate my birth or could we call it my re-birth.

In any event, it was much closer to becoming a daisy day and I not had seen too many of those in recent history.

Sunday came and went before I knew it. Then Monday came and the work would begin.

I had been given a schedule for both occupational and physical therapy—2 sessions in the morning and 2 in the afternoon.

Sometimes breakfast came late and all hell would break loose because everything and I mean EVERYTHING was now off schedule. I would still be hooked up to the feeding tube, trying to eat a limited breakfast, trying to get washed and dressed. An aide was coming to get me in five minutes to meet my therapists and take me by wheel chair to where ever I had to be fifteen minutes ago.

As I entered the huge room filled with exercise equipment, countless machines and other daily living devices, I was first amazed by the number of patients and secondly, the age which would range from 2 to 92. We had burn victims, strokes, knee replacements, hip replacements, birth defects and on and on. Oh, and me, I don't know what class I fell into but to quote one of my doctors, "He is alert, coherent, and appears emaciated. Manual muscle testing revealed fair strength in all extremities." The goals for my rehabilitation would be to: "improve strength, endurance, and ability to perform any mobility functions."

I guess we came to the right place.

During this same period, Dr. Joseph Hines, the extraordinary endocrinologist, was gracious enough to participate in my care while I was a patient at the rehab center. Of course, his expertise was treating my ongoing battle with diabetes.

My blood sugars were out of control, but what else would or could they be, based on the past few weeks.

Anyway, I was glad he showed and maintained an interest. I find him to be a very dedicated physician. Interested more in the patient and person than in processing numbers of any and all sort. I find him to be more of a "healer" than a "doctor."

I made it through day #1 of my therapies, but day #2 would be a different story. My blood sugars through the night were all over the chart and I was exhausted. The therapists gave me a respite, but we would make up for it in the days that followed.

I wish I could make the reader visualize in someway how this process continued. I can only use the comparison of a baby learning to walk. In this instance, however, you always had someone by your side or behind you. You would get on a bike, you would do tasks to strengthen your hands, arms and upper body. You would learn how to walk up and down a stairway, how to get up and down on a commode, and so on. It was back to basic training. If only my drill sergeant could see me now. "You want me to do how many push-ups?"

During this entire period, Chris was gathering information for medical review. In fact, both my primary care physician (Dr. Chrisman and also Dr. Hines) had someone on their staff doing research about my conditions.

In essence, both offices located basically the same information. Since there was no family history of any of these diseases, how did I get so lucky? Amazingly we would discover two studies that showed a linkage between pancreatic cancer and military service personnel exposed to Agent Orange while in Vietnam. Secondly, there was more evidence demonstrating a direct association between type II diabetes and Agent Orange exposure.

Chris initiated two applications; one for Social Security Disability and one with Veterans Affairs for service connected disability. Interesting in all of this was Chris was able to talk to Social Security. They asked her to see if she could get one of my physicians to fax them some additional needed information. She was successful, the doctors helped and the Social Security Administration found me to be disabled within a ten day period.

Strangely, I have not had that luck with Veterans Affairs. I can report that some decision of disability was made three years after the initial application dated March, 1999. Their

94

decision currently is under appeal as initiated by myself and my advocate through the American Legion located both in Erie and Washington, D.C.

This ongoing three year saga is a book unto itself.

Life was getting better! Days were getting longer! Spring was coming, but Valentine's Day was on the horizon first.

Days were daisier, if you know what I mean.

The diagnoses were there. The prognosis was guarded, but I was fighting back.

I really did know and I really did care!!! Thank God for my doctors. Thank God for the medical support staff. Thank God for family and friends. Thank God for prayer lines and for the people who will never know me, but still cared enough to pray for me.

Thank God for my best friend, my confidante, my cheerleader, my lover, my wife!!!

A few days before the arrival of Valentine's Day, I would have the honor to meet Dr. Mark Hogue, a clinical psychologist. I guess someone thought I needed some support services.

Dr. Hogue was a personable and likeable guy. He was a smooth talker and easy to talk to at the same time. My guess is that he was in the right business.

His findings were interesting, in as much as he found my surgeries, therapies, treatments and complications, "...reveals a likely picture of an adjustment disorder with depressed mood. Generally he had positive coping skills and has a history of being forward looking and positive regarding his life in general. He is understandably feeling quite overwhelmed at this time and, in fact, states that this word 'overwhelmed' better describes his emotions as opposed to 'depressed.' This is quite understandable at this time...His current plans are to increase his strength and endurance while here and he seems to have realistic plans." In some hand written notes, he states "...doubt meds will be needed. He's positive and forward-looking." I really liked this guy, but where the hell was he when I really needed him. Apparently, he didn't have an office on the same space ship as me.

I would have loved to have seen his notes about my hallucinations, delusions, and my psychotic state. Oh, well, just his luck!! He'll have to find someone else to write about in his own book.

While at Health South, Chris's uncle, Dr. Daniel C. Carnevale, an orthopedic surgeon of some stature would visit quite often. I was amazed at how much we actually conversed and he always was very positive, describing the need for me to be the same and to work diligently on regaining my strength.

Doctor Dan's wife, Sallie, would appear quite often. She was an Irish pixie, who enjoyed and relished life and still does. She and I have a special relationship as we always dance at family events to Frank Sinatra's version of "Start Spreading the News." For 70, she can still do a nasty high kick.

Whenever she came, she seemed to be spreading the news, the good news. She was a daisy-day maker.

Basic training continued and I continued to get stronger. After about a week I was able to shed the diapers. Just in time for my post-surgery visit back to Dr. Lee and Pittsburgh.

This event would take place on Friday, February 12, 1999. Initially, the social worker wanted my wife to drive me to and from Pittsburgh.

My advocate dug in her heels (she loves shoes) and said this plan was totally unacceptable. Her point was that I was still on insulin, a feeding tube, had difficulty with walking and bowel movements. How was she going to juggle all of this and drive the car too?

Ultimately, the rehab center director wrote an order for the need to be transported by ambulance.

At 9:00 a.m. on 2/12, two ambulance attendants appeared in my room. The plan was for me to be transported with necessary IV's sack lunch, insulin, etc. Within a short time, the attendants disappeared and so did the ambulance. I had a 1:30 p.m. appointment in Pittsburgh.

Subsequently, the ambulance attendants returned. However, they now had a registered nurse with them from the ambulance company. Apparently, they had no idea of my condition and that I needed a support system. They said the only way they could transport me would be with a nurse. We were running late—one driver and wife in front of ambulance—one ambulance attendant, registered nurse and patient in rear of ambulance. My wife could only say, "And they wanted me to drive you alone." She had made her point and would do so again with the social worker.

We flew to Pittsburgh faster than the "Spaceship Enterprise." OH! OH! Let's not go there.

The attendants said we wouldn't be in the doctor's office long. They don't like to have patients lying on stretchers in the middle of the waiting room.

We arrived at 1:10 p.m.   We were in an exam room at 1:15 p.m. We were seen at 1:20 p.m. We were on the road for a return to Erie no later than 2:15 p.m.   It was a long, exhausting day even without occupational or physical therapy.   As time progressed, so did I. Each morning now would include an inspection by the occupational therapist to verify that I had been able to dress myself.   I began to start eating more solid foods and could feel that some of my lost strength was returning. I was now able to get into my wheel chair unassisted; even to the point that I no longer needed an aide to push me down to physical therapy.   I became quite skilled at taking my feeding tube pole between my legs and wheeling down to therapy.   My days seemed to be getting a little bit daisier.

I continued on supplemental tube feedings. I continued to have vitals checked on a regular basis. My morning therapy sessions would be interrupted by blood sugar testing, dispensing of medications, insulin injections and the like.   Even my bowel movements had returned to normal. I know you really wanted to hear that.

Besides re-learning to walk, bend, sit, walk up and down stairs, and so on—I also had to learn how to seat myself in a car as both a driver and passenger.   I never knew how involved something could be. On one occasion, a fellow patient and I were going through and being put through our paces in reference to getting in and out of a car. A partial model of a real car was in the building and on this particular day, I was playing the role of passenger.   I reached over and tried to honk the horn and told my fellow patient, Joe, to get us the hell out of here.   Needless to say, there was no battery for the horn to work and Joe and I knew; we weren't going anywhere.

I have to admit that the staff at this facility was most gracious, efficient and caring. I can only recall one incident that was of concern to me.

As you know, my blood sugars were tested regularly and always at 3:00 a.m. If I was in need of insulin, I would receive an injection as prescribed.

One particular 3:00 a.m. visit brought a male nurse into my room. He took my blood sugar and I asked him what it was because I felt shaky and was sweating. He replied that my blood sugar level was 53 and he would return with my insulin injection.

I began to protest and said I was not going to be given an injection. The nurse replied that he had to give me this shot because my chart said an insulin injection was given at this time.

Once again I protested and said that I had the right to refuse medication. I explained that if he gave me an injection at this point, he would lower my blood sugar level to a critical area that could put me into a coma. I instructed him to get me a glass of orange juice and return in another hour to retake my blood sugar. He did so and an hour later my sugars were at 130 or 140 so that he could use the insulin.

I wonder how many other cases like this took place with different results.

In any event, as I said, the staff and care provided at this facility would have to be classified as close to excellent.

By the end of week two, I was ready for an overnight pass. I would get to come home for a short spell to see if I could manage on my own.

We quickly learned that while I could seat myself on a commode; I was unable to get up unassisted. Secondly, I had difficulty in using stairs (both up and down.) We brought this information back so that we knew what areas we had to continue to work on and we did.

But, oh my, how nice it was to see the inside of our home. We had a number of visitors, but I was still amazed at how quickly I tired.

Upon return to the facility, I would return to my therapy with a new passion and zest. I wanted out of here—I wanted to go home.

I would get another over-night pass and would do much better the following week. Ultimately, my wife and advocate insisted on a staffing relative to my case. She wanted assurances that I could not only go home, but be self-sufficient because I would be alone most of the day.

Every staff person was very positive about my performance and my progress. However, they agreed to spend the next couple of days putting me through my paces. The paces were multiple and difficult, but we made it.

I was about to get ready to make the great escape. Chris had purchased chocolates for the nursing staff on my floor, the social worker, and occupational and physical therapists in partial gratitude for their dedication and attention to my case. I can only be forever grateful to a group of caring people.

I'm going home Baby!!! This is the daisiest of days in a very long time. It's still snowing, but all I can see are daisies.

CHAPTER 17

Home Again

It was the ending of February and the beginning of March and I would finally get my "marching" papers in order to make the great escape.

I was going home, again. In spite of what the great American author, Thomas Wolfe, said, "You can't go home again!"

The ride was comfortable and uneventful as we drove south from Erie to Meadville on the Interstate. It was just gratifying to see different scenery and more gratifying to see scenery at all.

We would arrive home by mid-afternoon. Within an hour of our arrival, both the visiting nurses' representative and a physical therapist would appear on the doorstep.

The first actions of the visiting nurse was to do some checking of my vital signs. Next, she would determine if I could get up and down stairs and in or out of the bathtub/shower.

The most interesting part of her visit was the inspection of my open wound. She would measure the length and width and make other observations. Next, she would remove the dressing and instruct both Chris and I how to apply fresh dressings twice a day.

I must admit this was not a pretty picture nor was it a pleasing exercise. Nonetheless, it was something that had to be done. I had to avoid infection and insure that the healing process would take place.

We would be left sufficient supplies to cover the next couple of days until a medical services supplier could make a home delivery. Before the visiting nurse left, the physical therapist appeared. The purpose of the visit was basically to determine if I needed a therapist in the home to provide me with therapy and instruction or could I do this on my own with written instruction.

For the next hour or so, the therapist put me through my paces. Doing leg lifts in various positions, doing lifts with hand and ankle weights, standing on one foot, and on and on.

As it turned out, I was a quick learner and a compliant patient.

I wanted to get better! I wanted to get stronger!

The decision was made that I could achieve what I needed to without close supervision or instruction. I knew what I had to do, how to do it, how many times, at what intervals, etc.

Finally, Chris and I were beginning to settle in for my first initial and official night home. Of course, part of that regimen would be to hook up to my old friend "Herman."

It was interesting how we didn't forget or miss a beat on how to hook up old faithful. Unfortunately, I had been gone so long that as time progressed the feeding tube would shut down and off every hour. Needless to say, this became quite annoying. Before long, Chris and I were on the phone with the supplier to find out what we were doing wrong.

We were walked through all the steps over the phone. As it turned out, there needed to be some re-programming of the device since I had been absent and off this machine for nearly two months while I was hospitalized and in the rehabilitation center.

Strangely, we were successful in getting this machine to do what it needed to do so that we could get down to the important business at hand.

SLEEP! QUIET, PEACEFUL, NO INTERRUPTIONS, RESTFUL SLEEP.

It had been a long and eventful day!!

The next few months would be filled with a multitude of medical events.

The refrigerator door began to reflect my itinerary of which doctor I would see, when and where. I really needed a secretary to keep track of all these appointments.

Namely who would or could take me where or when. In addition to these appointments, I would be required to visit "Count Dracula" on a regular basis to determine how things were going or weren't going as the case might be.

The doctors' visits included my primary care physician, surgeon, specialists—you name it. I was beginning to think some of these places could name a wing of their building after me or at least, put up a plaque, "I had been here."

The visiting nurse continued to visit at least twice a week. The open wound would be measured at each visit. It was getting better and smaller. There would be less and less drainage and blood. We were doing the dressing changes correctly. There were no signs of infection.

I was getting better! I was getting stronger! I wasn't getting fatter. But, hey, two out of three ain't bad.

103

Finally, there would come a time in May that I could speak to both my surgeons and primary care physician. It was time for me to make my case.

I had to get off this feeding tube!!

The continuous whining noise of the liquid being forced through the tube by the machine and ultimately into my body was beginning to drive me up the wall.

"Herman" continued to hold me hostage in our own den on the couch. I needed a sense of freedom. I was back on a regular diet with an appetite. While I continued not to gain an appreciable amount of weight. I was able to maintain a level.

I finally convinced those who needed convincing that I could and would survive without the efforts of "Herman."

In mid-May, I would pay a visit to my primary care physician. The feeding tube would be removed. The hole would be covered by bandages for some time, but it, too, like the open wound would heal from the inside out and I could function again without a space-like hook-up. I would be "free to move about the cabin", unencumbered and untethered.

I would be free to sleep in my own bed after an absence of over nine months. It would be nice to have a warm, loving body next to mine.

It was good to be home!

It was good to be stronger!

It was good to be better!

It was good to be free!

Life was good!!!

The days were getting daisier! The flowers were in bloom!

CHAPTER 18

Some Tough Decisions

It was still early spring, but I would soon be forced to make some very difficult decisions.

I continued to use my sick days from employment as I had accrued over 250 days over my years of service with the State government. These days were earned at 13 days per year and since I had been pretty healthy prior to my current encounters, I was able to save a great number of days. In essence, it was somewhat like an insurance policy and I'm happy to say, "a damn good one."

Based on tests, treatments, exams, diagnosis, prognosis, and so on—I needed to make some hard and tough decisions.

Should I take disability retirement?

Should I take early retirement?

There were many options to weigh. If I chose disability, my wife and other heirs, would essentially be left with nothing. Some additional financial penalties/losses would occur.

By some stroke of luck (if you can call it that) I qualified for early retirement with full payment and benefits because I met both age qualifications and number of years of service. The greatest benefit of this option was the lack of penalties for taking early retirement and the ability for your heirs to inherit something without being penalized.

The bottom line here required me to discuss my situation not only with a retirement counselor but also an accountant.

More importantly, there was a need to discuss this situation (my situation) in greater depth with the medical community responsible for my care and ongoing treatment. Did I have more questions than answers—you bet. Were the answers as clear and concise as I wanted them to be—never.

There is just so much to think about. If I do this, am I giving up? If I do that, am I sealing my fate? What to do? What to do?

To complicate matters regarding early retirement, the current legislation allowing early retirement with no penalties would end on June 30, 1999. Bottom line, you had to decide to retire before that date or the window of opportunity would close.

Now, could I take my chances and wait for another opportunity to come along? I guess so, but the way opportunities were showing up on my doorstep these days led me to believe that there wouldn't be too many coming our way.

Between having my feeding tube removed and a colonoscopy tube inserted, I would decide that it was time. Time to decide. Time to take early retirement.

Strangely, through all of this, Chris was intent on the creation of a rock garden that she wanted built on the south side of our home.

We had talked about this for some time and I guess I would always say the right things to placate her or put her off as long as I could.

She had spent most of this spring researching where she could purchase the right rocks and at the right price. She would also need top soil, sand and so on. Costs were beginning to mount.

On the day I returned from a colonoscopy, I was utterly amazed and dumbfounded to see a tri-axle truck appear in our driveway. I ran and I mean ran from the front door of our house to the back to tell my wife: "Did you see this thing? Did you see this truck? Did you see the load it's carrying? Did you know about this?"

In a calming tone and voice, Chris was more than aware that this truck was coming. What I don't think she was aware of was that we were about to get enough stones to build the Church of the Holy Sepulcher. If not a church, at least, a small chapel.

Before all was said and done, it was determined that neither she or I were able to move these stones either independently or in concert with each other.

We had paid $150.00 for the stones, five times as many as we needed. We would soon learn that we would need someone to design and create this rock garden—some additional costs. Oh, yeah!

I think this rock garden after all the additional costs would quickly approach over $1,000.00. Happy Mother's Day! Happy Birthday! Merry Christmas! Happy Easter!

To add to this, we still had enough stones to complete our chapel. We would invite family, friends, neighbors, and yes, even strangers, to please take a rock home with you.

I was convinced I needed to retire. Someone had to stay home and protect the integrity of the home fires, the checkbook, the surrounding land, and so on.

But I was getting stronger!

I would submit my letter of resignation and intent to retire as required.

Paperwork, paperwork, paperwork!!!

The retirement counselor was gracious enough to come to my home on two or three occasions in order to get this accomplished.

I would attend my last official manager's meeting in Harrisburg and be pleasantly surprised by a retirement dinner. Included was a citation from the State Legislature for my years of service, which I felt very humbled and gratified by during the evening's festivities. It had been a wonderful run—33 years of credited service!!! I would miss it all!!

I would be feted later in the month of June in Erie by my local office and by friends and colleagues from former places of employment. Other friends and family members would attend.

It was good to see so many people and to hear so many stories.

LIFE WAS GOOD...

CHAPTER 19

Tests and Treatments

June was a glorious month too, because a dear friend married his dear friend after a lengthy courtship (and I mean lengthy). Andy Stofan's wife has the staying power of a fully equipped space ship. If she even heard the words, "Houston, we have a problem," she would deal with it so fast your head would spin.

In any event, I got to travel to the Latrobe area (home of Arnold Palmer and Rolling Rock Beer) to celebrate the grand occasion. I swear it must have been 98 degrees in the shade for the out door wedding ceremony. At some point, I think we all wished that there was a keg of beer for each side of the artificial aisle.

My wife and I enjoyed the good times with good friends. Friends that had supported us through this year long (out-of-body) experience.

As we drove away from the Latrobe area at noon, we headed for a private home. Chris had directions and she wanted me to see something. Little did I know that my belated Father's Day gift awaited me.

As we arrived at the home of this mid-30's aged couple, we were greeted by two female puppies—Boxer puppies.

I had been talking about getting a companion to help me in my rehabilitation process and wanted to replace our former Boxer, who had to be put down due to cancer almost two years prior.

Of course, I immediately fell in love with both pups, but I became transfixed by the mouthy, independent one.

She seemed to enjoy playing hide and seek and was intent on giving me a run for my money.

Thus, I would be the final judge in deciding which pup would make the two and half hour return trip home and become a permanent part of our family circle.

The decision was made. No docile, quiet pup for me. She would have to be someone, who could communicate her wants and needs and so the choice was simple.

She rode home most of the way, asleep in my lap. A few whimpers from time to time, one stop for nature and a return to her nest.

As we drove into our driveway, our pup awoke and seemed to be aware that she was home. And so, "Mr. P's Renaissance Lady", or Rennie as she would become known, had arrived.

She, indeed, was part of a treatment plan!! Little did I know how much this eight week old pup would begin to insist how much more I needed to do in order to be a part of her active life.

During the next several months, both Chris and I would continue our ongoing schedule of tests, treatments (if needed), medications and change in medications, fasting and non-fasting tests and on and on.

The refrigerator continued to be covered with two sheets of paper, one for each of us. Each sheet would cover a two or three-month interval in which appointments had been scheduled with physicians or certain tests would have to be performed by specific dates.

Fall would come quickly and would begin in earnest my desire to plant hundred of spring bulbs to herald in a re-birth, a renaissance (if you will) of our lives, our renewed lives.

The season would also bring training for Rennie. I'm not sure if I took her to school or she took me, but she is one very smart dog. She would pass with flying colors. I, on the other hand, was not the best handler in the world. However, Rennie accepted my short comings and ultimately, we graduated from the course.

Fall would also bring a return to the Cancer Institute in Pittsburgh. I continued as a participant of the study group for the use of a vaccine. At this time, I was eligible for what was known as a "Booster", which is given on an annual basis.

I would first have two vials of blood drawn to see if I could continue through the process. I would then be seen by Dr. Ramanathan, who continued to conduct the study. This visit would encompass vitals and a physical exam, which spent a great deal of time checking lymph node areas, as well as, the area of initial determination of the cancer—pancreas, stomach, liver and so on.

I was pleased to hear him say that of all the participants, my immune system kicked in the most positively.

I was cleared to go to the treatment floor. Again, I would have blood drawn—only this time "Count Dracula" needed six vials. As I understand it, certain tests had to be conducted, which ultimately determined the make-up, mixture and strength of the booster injection.

As I said before, this would become a day-long event. We would leave for Pittsburgh at 8:00 a.m. and return home about 6:00 p.m.

111

Nonetheless, we got the shot and an arm that ached for the next 24 to 36 hours with accompanying flu-like symptoms.

But—it was worth it! I was convinced this vaccine was having a positive impact in extending my life!!

Chris would continue to have labs and MRIs. At the same time, I would continue with labs, CAT scans, colonoscopies and other exams.

We continued to need to locate someone to help us keep track of all these appointments.

Fall continued and the bulb planting in concert with the season. The only bulbs not planted were those that Rennie stole and she would either not return or I could not retrieve. I'm convinced there's a beautiful spring garden somewhere in the nearby woods.

Life was good!! Days of Daisies began to outnumber Days of Barbed Wire!

CHAPTER 20

The Long, Long Road

The period between Christmas, 1999, and the present were filled with much of the same.

Chris continues to have regular exams, lab work and so on. She continues to be treated for high blood pressure, high cholesterol and diabetes. Her medications are oral and she averages a dozen pills per day.

I, too, continue with a regimen of tests, exams, lab work and treatment. I continue to remain on numerous medications for anemia, ulcerative colitis, diabetes and pancreatic cancer. Oral medications number in the area of thirty per day plus three insulin injections.

The road has been long; the road has been winding. More importantly, there still is a road.

We were blessed to learn on Christmas Eve, 2000, that our numbers would be increased by the birth of our first grandchild.

Abigail Lynn made her appearance on August 13, 2001. She is and has been a gift from God.

She fits nicely into and between our scheduled medical appointments. She is a joy to behold! Of course, I'm convinced all grandparents say and think that. But it is so great to be able to spoil her.

On Mother's Day, 2001, I gave my daughter-in-law a special gift for the not yet born, Abigail. Her mom would be the keeper of Abby's first pair of diamond earrings.

Some people think I'm nuts, but I want her to know I was here and I was thinking about her.

She is a bouquet of daisies!!!

The road continues with unknown valleys, curves, hills, pot-holes and the like. But—the road continues and life _is_ good!!!

CHAPTER 21

Meet the Dream Team

I'd like to introduce you to current and past members of what I call the "Dream Team." People, who have come together in various ways, in order to treat me and allow the road (or have some part in it) to continue.

Dr. R. Bruce Dratler—diagnosed ulcerative colitis in May, 1996. Continues to provide care and treatment. There is "no end in sight" in his job.

Dr. LeAnne Chrisman—diagnosed diabetes, type II in March, 1998. —diagnosed pancreatic cancer in July, 1998. Probably, single-handedly, prolonged or saved my life. Now practicing in the Cleveland, Ohio area.

Dr. Wolfgang Schroat—performed Whipple Procedure in July, 1998. Continues to provide follow-up care as needed.

Dr. Kenneth Lee—performed first and second surgeries for bowel perforation in 1999. Continues to provide follow-up care, testing and treatment.

Dr. Joseph Hines—took over treatment of diabetes in October, 1998. He has followed me since and hopefully, will never leave my side.

Dr. David D. Howell, Jr.—radiologist/oncologist at Regional Cancer Center, who was smart enough to recommend no radiation in my case. Now practicing in Indianapolis, Indiana.

Dr. Aiman Dhaghestani—oncologist, who was the first physician to <u>really</u> explain my prognosis. Over saw my chemotherapy treatments and is now practicing in the Detroit, Michigan area.

Dr. Ramesh Ramanathan ——--- research oncologist and lead person for the continued testing of the vaccine, Muscin.

Dr. Conrado Toledano—Director of Health South Rehabilitation Hospital. Over saw and directed my care and treatment.

Dr. Robert Schwartz—a gifted gastro-enterologist, who I came to know at the Rehabilitation Center. The Center's Director had sought a consultation with him and through his efforts; he got me back to some normalcy. Strikes me as a very knowledgeable and bright guy. Unfortunately, have not seen or talked to him since my release from Health South.

Dr. Mark Hogue—clinical psychologist, who was smart enough to know that I knew when and if I needed him; he would be there.

116

Dr. Jack Peterson—primary care physician for both Chris and me since September, 2000. Very thorough, very bright, attentive listener and a very caring practitioner.

Dr. Edward J. Miskiel—oncologist on loan to local Regional Cancer Center, who I met in February, 2002. Dr. Miskiel had previous experience at both the West Virginia Veterans' Administration and Togus, Maine Veterans' facilities. He was kind enough to write the Department of Veterans' Affairs for me. He wrote in part, "...there is no doubt in my mind that the patient's exposure to Agent Orange was the cause of this patient's bizarre malignancy."

I had planned to list everyone else who has provided both Chris and I with their support. Unfortunately, every time I would list one name, I would find that I had forgotten three.

In an effort to avoid slighting anyone, I am going to recognize everyone in concert:

- All medical and support staff

- All family members

- All friends

- All prayer-line individuals

- All ministers and their ministries

- All medical supply providers

- Anyone and everyone

117

Finally,

Chris Palotas—my best friend, my lover, my confidante, my wife, my cheerleader, my advocate.   Without her tenacity, I would not be here today. I am forever grateful.

The Dream Team worked as a well oiled machine. Working in concert with each other and not individually in a vacuum of self-importance.

CHAPTER 22

So Why This Book?

Call it cathartic, therapeutic, a voice shouting in my ear.
Call it anything you like.
From our stand point, Chris knows that her tumor could easily return within ten years of its removal.
As far as me, most pancreatic cancers return within eighteen months, less than 4 percent of pancreatic patients survive in excess of five years.
We indeed have been and are blessed.
And so I guess I want to further say:

I can—I can't

I will—I won't

I did—I didn't

I could—I couldn't

I should—I shouldn't

I would—I wouldn't
and so on.

All the foregoing are actions, some positive and others negative. My history and military training leads me to believe and be convinced that nothing is impossible— nothing!!

I read somewhere recently that it is a bad attitude that can be the cause of a disability.

My goals in all of this bantering follow:

- Bring some shared hope and knowledge to others.

- Bring some laughter into someone's heart.

- Bring a change in the Cancer Society's position on survivors. It is critical that we recognize all those who have been part of the struggle as equals.

- Bring about empty parking lots at Regional Cancer Centers.

- Bring about "for sale/lease/rent" signs on every Cancer Center.

- Bring about an understanding that cancer patients are not contagious.

- Bring about some daisies for all the rest of your days.

Those who know me personally (and know me well) are aware that I love Broadway musicals. In particular, anything done by Mr. Andrew Lloyd Weber. I am particularly drawn to one of the songs that appears in the first act of The Phantom of the Opera. As my wife (Christine) knows, I am both her Phantom and Raoul. I believe all of us who have in some way shared in this experience would want everyone who knows them to know the following:

"Think of me, think of me fondly when we say good-bye.
Remember me—once in awhile.
Please promise me you'll try.

When you find that once again you long to take your heart back and be free
If you ever find a moment—spare a thought for me.

We never said our love was evergreen
or as unchanging as the sea

But, if you can still remember—
stop and think of me.

Think of all the things we've shared and seen
Don't think about the things which might have been.

Think of me, think of me waking silent and resigned.
Imagine me trying too hard to put you from my mind
Recall those days, look back on all those times.

Think of the things we'll never do.

There will never be a day when
I won't think of you.

We never said our love was ever-green
or as unchanging as the sea.

But, please promise me that
sometimes, you will think of me!"

And so, we continue.

CHAPTER 23

In the Beginning

I refuse to allow this book to say "The End."

Everyday is a new beginning.

Everyday is a chance at re-birth.

Everyday is a renaissance.

Everyday is a new challenge.

Everyday is a celebration.

And so, there is no ending in sight. Just an endless amount of new beginnings.

Days filled with daisies.

Days filled with barbed-wire.

Days filled with daisies and barbed-wire.

And life—life is good!!!